Progress in
Cancer Research and Therapy
Volume 24

RECENT CLINICAL DEVELOPMENTS
IN GYNECOLOGIC ONCOLOGY

Progress in Cancer Research and Therapy

Progress in
Cancer Research and Therapy
Volume 24

Recent Clinical Developments in Gynecologic Oncology

Editors

C. Paul Morrow, M.D.
Director of Gynecologic Oncology
Department of Obstetrics and Gynecology
University of Southern California
School of Medicine
Women's Hospital
Los Angeles, California

John Bonnar, M.A., M.D., F.R.C.O.G.
Department of Obstetrics and Gynaecology
University of Dublin
Trinity College Unit
Totunda Hospital
Dublin, Ireland

Timothy J. O'Brien, Ph.D.
Division of Gynecologic Oncology
Department of Obstetrics and Gynecology
University of Southern California
School of Medicine
Women's Hospital
Los Angeles, California

William E. Gibbons, M.D.
Division of Endocrinology
Department of Obstetrics and Gynecology
University of Southern California
School of Medicine
Women's Hospital
Los Angeles, California
Presently: Baylor University
School of Medicine
Houston, Texas

Raven Press ■ New York

Raven Press, 1140 Avenue of the Americas, New York, New York 10036

Made in the United States of America

Library of Congress Cataloging in Publication Data
Main entry under title:

Recent clinical developments in gynecologic oncology.
    (Progress in cancer research and therapy ; v. 24)
    Includes bibliographies and index.
    1. Generative organs, Female—Cancer—Addresses,
essays, lectures.   I. Morrow, C. Paul (Charles Paul)
[DNLM: 1. Genital neoplasms, Female. W1 PR667M v.24/
WP 145 R294]
RC280.G5R43   1983   616.99'465   83-3312
ISBN 0-89004-810-X

Preface

The focus of this volume is on the changes taking place in the diagnosis and management of gynecologic cancer and related conditions. The topics addressed cover many important areas of progress and controversy occurring in the field of gynecologic cancer in the past ten years. Readers will find a very selective, problem-oriented format by international experts intended to put into perspective the development of the past decade in terms of optimal current therapy and assessment.

The first chapter by Lavery and Pinkerton proposes that vulvar lichen sclerosus is etiologically related to diabetes mellitus and other endocrine disturbances. The arguments suggest new approaches to therapy. In the following chapter, Duncan presents the results of his experience with the Semm "cold" coagulator (operates at 100°C), which may be superior to the cryosurgical method of ablating cervical dysplasia. Fox discusses the perennial problems of gynecologic pathology, atypical endometrial hyperplasia, and borderline ovarian tumors. One of the world's experts on hormone receptors, Professor Griffiths of Cardiff and co-workers, discuss the relationship of hormone receptors to treatment and outcome in breast cancer. The chapters by Gibbons and O'Brien, and Soutter et al. present new data on hormone receptors in malignancies of the female pelvis.

The chapters in this volume consider other topics of current interest in gynecologic oncology including new data on periaortic node irradiation in cervical cancer (Kolstad); venous thromboembolism (Bonnar); surgical staging of endometrial carcinoma; and a simplified clonogenic assay (Sykes et al.); laparoscopy; and the management of intractable cancer pain. The final chapter deals with care of the terminal cancer patient.

This book will be of practical importance to gynecologists, gynecologic oncologists, and other specialists who deal with pelvic neoplasms in women.

C. Paul Morrow, M.D.
John Bonnar, M.D.
Timothy J. O'Brien, Ph.D.
William E. Gibbons, M.D.

Dedication

This book contains a series of original papers presented at a conference on gynecologic cancer held at Trinity College Dublin, September 1–3, 1981. This conference was organized to honor James F. Nolan, one of the outstanding gynecologic oncologists in the United States, at the time of his retirement from active practice. His accomplishments set him apart as a scientist, inventor, and teacher.

After receiving his doctorate from the Washington University School of Medicine, St. Louis, in 1938, Dr. Nolan took his residency training in obstetrics and gynecology at the St. Louis Maternity Hospital under Professors Willard M. Allen and Axel N. Arneson. His next year was spent with Edith Quimby at the Memorial Hospital in New York City as a special fellow of the National Cancer Institute (1942–1943).

This unusual background of training in obstetrics-gynecology and radiation medicine resulted in his assignment as Post Surgeon at Los Alamos, New Mexico during the development of the atom bomb. He served as the scientific courier aboard the ill-fated USS Indianapolis which delivered the first atom bomb to the island of Tinian in the Marianas. Dr. Nolan was a member of the team of Americans entering Japan to evaluate the effects of the atom bombs dropped on Nagasaki and Hiroshima. Later he participated as a consultant to the Atomic Energy Commission during the atom bomb testing at Eniwetok and Bikini.

After leaving the military service in 1946, Dr. Nolan served on the faculty of the Washington University School of Medicine for two years before entering private practice in Los Angeles, California. In this setting, Dr. Nolan and a physicist friend, Russell H. Neil, constructed one of the first cobalt teletherapy units to be used for cancer treatment in the United States. He later designed a radium applicator system for cervical cancer utilizing ovoid colpostats fixed to an adjustable uterine tandem. With a teaching appointment at the Los Angeles County-University of Southern California Medical Center, Dr. Nolan was in charge of the gynecologic tumor service for many years. This teaching post brought to him a clinical professorship in both gynecology and radiation therapy.

During his distinguished career, Dr. Nolan has contributed over 40 publications to the literature on gynecologic cancer concerned primarily with the treatment of cervical and endometrial cancer. He is a member of eleven national medical societies including the prestigious American Gynecological Society, the American Association of Obstetricians and Gynecologists, and the Society of Pelvic Surgeons. He has served as President of the American Radium Society, the Los Angeles Society of Obstetricians and Gynecologists and the Western Association of Gynecologic Oncologists, a society whose existence is a monument to his stature in the community of gynecologic oncologists.

Contents

Contributors

R. W. Blamey, M.D.
The City Hospital
Nottingham, NG5 1PB England

John Bonnar, M.A., M.D.,
F.R.C.O.G.
Department of Obstetrics and
*   Gynaecology*
University of Dublin
Trinity College Unit
Rotunda Hospital
Dublin 1, Ireland

C. Campbell, M.D.
The City Hospital
Nottingham, NG5 1PB England

J. J. Campbell, M.D.
Peter MacCallum Hospital
Melbourne, Australia

Ian D. Duncan, M.B., Ch.B.,
M.R.O.C.G.
Department of Obstetrics and Gynecology
Ninewells Hospital and Medical School
Dundee DD1 9SY, Scotland

J. J. Fennelly, M.D., F.R.C.P.I.
St. Vincent's Hospital and National
*   Maternity Hospital*
Elm Park
Dublin, Ireland

H. Fox, M.D.
Department of Pathology
Stopford Building
University of Manchester
Oxford Road
Manchester M13 9PT, England

William E. Gibbons, M.D.
Department of Obstetrics and Gynecology
Baylor University School of Medicine
Houston, Texas 77027

R. W. Green-Thompson, M.B.,
Ch.B., M.R.C.O.G.,
F.C.O.G. (SA)
Department of Gynaecology
Faculty of Medicine
University of Natal
Durban, Republic of South Africa

K. Griffiths, Ph.D.
Tenovus Institute for Cancer Research
Cardiff, CF4 4XN Wales

S. M. Joubert, M.Sc., F.R.C.
Path.
Department of Chemical Pathology
Faculty of Medicine
University of Natal
Durban, Republic of South Africa

B. Joyce, Ph.D.
Tenovus Institute for Cancer Research
Cardiff, CF4 4XN Wales

Per Kolstad, M.D.,
F.R.C.O.G. (Hon)
Department of Gynecology
The Norwegian Radium Hospital
Montebello, Oslo 3, Norway

Conley G. Lacey, M.D.
Department of Obstetrics and Gynecology
University of California, San Francisco
350 Parnassus Avenue
San Francisco, California 94117

Hilary A. Lavery, M.D.
Department of Midwifery and
  Gynaecology
The Queen's University of Belfast
Grosvenor Road
Belfast BT 12 6BJ, Northern Ireland

Patrick Finian Lynch, M.D.,
  B.Ch., B.A.O., M.R.C.O.G.
Coombe Lying-in Hospital
Dublin, Ireland

C. Paul Morrow, M.D.
Department of Obstetrics and Gynecology
University of Southern California School
  of Medicine
Women's Hospital
1240 North Mission Road
Los Angeles, California 90033

M. Morton, Ph.D.
Tenovus Institute for Cancer Research
Cardiff, CF4 4XN Wales

R. Murray, M.D., F.R.A.C.P.
Peter MacCallum Hospital and Endocrine
  Clinic
Cancer Institute
University of Melbourne
Melbourne, Australia

D. V. Naidoo, M.B., Ch.B.
Department of Gynaecology
Faculty of Medicine
University of Natal
Durban, Republic of South Africa

R. I. Nicholson, Ph.D.
Tenovus Institute for Cancer Research
Cardiff, CF4 4XN Wales

James F. Nolan, M.D.,
  F.A.C.O.G., F.A.C.S.
Departments of Obstetrics and
  Gynecology and Radiology
Southern California Cancer Center
1414 South Hope Street
Los Angeles, California 90015

Timothy J. O'Brien, Ph.D.
Division of Gynecologic Oncology
Department of Obstetrics and Gynecology
University of Southern California School
  of Medicine
Women's Hospital
1240 North Mission Road
Los Angeles, California 90033

Michael J. O'Halloran, M.D.,
  F.F.R.I., F.R.C.R.
Saint Luke's Hospital
Highfield Road
Rathgar, Dublin 6, Ireland

R. J. Pegoraro, B.Sc.
Department of Chemical Pathology
Faculty of Medicine
University of Natal
Durban, Republic of South Africa

R. J. Pepperell, M.D.
Department of Obstetrics and
  Gynaecology
University of Melbourne
Melbourne, Australia

R. H. Philpott, M.D., F.R.C.O.G.
Department of Gynaecology
Faculty of Medicine
University of Natal
Durban, Republic of South Africa

John H. M. Pinkerton, M.D.
Department of Midwifery and
  Gynaecology
The Queen's University of Belfast
Grosvenor Road
Belfast BT 12 6BJ, Northern Ireland

M. A. Quinn, M.D.
Department of Obstetrics and
  Gynaecology
University of Melbourne
Melbourne, Australia

Hugh Raftery, M.D., B.Ch.,
B.A.O., F.F.A., R.C.S.I.
St. Laurence's Hospital
43 Rathdown Park
Terenure Dublin 6, Ireland

John B. Schlaerth, M.D.
Department of Obstetrics and Gynecology
University of Southern California School
of Medicine
Women's Hospital
1240 North Mission Road
Los Angeles, California 90033

W. P. Soutter, M.D., M.Sc.,
M.R.C.O.G.
Department of Obstetrics and
Gynaecology
University of Sheffield
The Jessop Hospital for Women
Sheffield S3 7RE, England

John A. Sykes, M.D.
Southern California Cancer Center
1414 South Hope Street
Los Angeles, California 90015

Recent Clinical Developments in Gynecologic Oncology, edited by C. Paul Morrow, et al. Raven Press, New York © 1983.

Vulval Dystrophy: Its Aetiology and Classification

Hilary A. Lavery and John H. M. Pinkerton

Department of Midwifery and Gynaecology, The Queen's University of Belfast, Belfast BT12 6BJ, Northern Ireland

Pruritus (itching) of the vulva is a common and often intractable condition in older women. It may be associated with obvious skin lesions, such as moniliasis and psoriasis, which if accurately diagnosed can usually be effectively treated. However, pruritus associated with ill-defined and variable changes in the vulval skin, for which no specific cause is apparent, is much more difficult to manage. In the past, various terms usually derived from the clinical appearances have been used to describe such nonspecific changes; more recently, the term "vulval dystrophy" has been suggested to describe all such vulval lesions, whether red or white, thickened or atrophic, which can be further classified according to their detailed histological appearance. A review of the literature shows how a more satisfactory nomenclature and classification system has gradually evolved.

LEUKOPLAKIA

According to Sir Comyns Berkeley and Victor Bonney (1) of the Middlesex Hospital in London, the term "leukoplakia," which is derived from the Greek *leukos* (white) and *plax* (plate), was coined in 1869 by Hulke to describe certain oral lesions. It became firmly established in the gynaecological literature in 1909, when Berkeley and Bonney defined leukoplakic vulvitis as a chronic inflammatory disease that was invariably premalignant (this aspect will be dealt with later) affecting the labia majora and minora, perineum, perianal region, and thighs. The vestibule and urethra were never, they believed, affected. They described four clinical and four uncorrelated histological stages of the condition (Table 1).

In 1929, Taussig (15) of the United States held that leukoplakic vulvitis could affect any part of the vulval skin, from the mons veneris to the anus. However, in 6 of his 40 patients only the perineum and the perianal areas were involved. The early clinical appearance was characterized by reddish grey and thickened skin, which later became white and parchment-like. Taussig recognized only two microscopic stages (Table 2). Like Berkeley and Bonney, he believed that leukoplakia always progressed to carcinoma. The meaning of leukoplakia was thus altered from its original connotation of simply white plaque to carry a more sinister implication

1

TABLE 1. *Clinical and histological stages of leukoplakic vulvitis*

Stage	Manifestations
Clinical stage	
1	Reddening, swelling, excoriation, dryness
2	Subepithelial thickening of labia majora, thinning of labia minora, semiopaque and white areas of skin
3	Cracks, ulceration, bleeding, carcinoma
4	Smooth, white, shiny skin atrophy of labia minora and clitoris
Histological stage[a]	
1	Swollen epithelium, lymphocytic infiltrates
2	Dermal infiltrate of lymphocytes and plasma cells, subepithelial homogenous zone, loss of elastic tissue
3	Fibrosis, disappearance of inflammatory cells, absence of elastic tissue
4	Sclerosus complete

[a]Note that histological stages do not correspond to clinical stages.
From Berkeley and Bonner (1).

TABLE 2. *Stages of leukoplakic vulvitis*

Stage 1. Hypertrophic stage (reddish grey skin)
   Parakeratosis
   Hyperkeratosis
   Acanthosis
   Lymphocytic infiltration of corium
Stage 2. Atrophic stage (white skin)
   Hyperkeratosis
   Epidermal atrophy
   Subepithelial collagenous zone
   Chronic inflammatory cell infiltration of the corium

From Taussig (15).

of precancerous white plaque. The more recent practice of some authors, e.g., McAdams and Kistner (13), of using the term leukoplakia to describe conditions in which there is histological evidence of atypia irrespective of the gross appearance has only further confused the issue. In the past, clinicians, understandably reluctant to diagnose leukoplakia, which they had been taught implied premalignancy and for which the treatment was vulvectomy, biopsied such vulval lesions in the hope that the pathologist would determine if the condition was indeed leukoplakia. Pathologists, however, were unwilling to use this term at all, since they considered it to be a purely clinical description; historically and etymologically this is correct.

KRAUROSIS VULVAE

The term kraurosis vulvae first appeared in the literature when used by Breisky (2) in 1885. Contrary to common belief, kraurosis, which is derived from the Greek *kraurosis* (brittle), does not mean shrinkage. Breisky originally used the term to describe a condition of progressive atrophy affecting the labia majora and minora in which the skin became shiny, dry, and white. He recognized only one stage. Clinically and histologically the appearance is essentially identical with Taussig's second or atrophic stage of leukoplakic vulvitis (Table 2). There is little agreement among subsequent authors on the precise relationship between kraurosis and leukoplakic vulvitis (Table 3).

TABLE 3. *Relationship of kraurosis vulvae to leukoplakic vulvitis*

Separate entity from leukoplakic vulvitis [Berkeley and Bonney (1)]
End stage of 50% of cases of leukoplakia [Taussig (15)]
Progresses to leukoplakia in 10 yr in 50% [Wallace and Whimster (16)]

LICHEN SCLEROSUS

It 1889, the dermatologist Hallopeau (8) described an atrophic skin lesion that he believed to be a late stage of lichen planus as lichen planus atrophicus. Subsequently, this became known as lichen sclerosus et (or vel) atrophicus and, more recently, as lichen sclerosus. Macroscopically, the typical lesions are white polygonal papules, which progress to atrophic parchment-like plaques. The extragenital areas usually affected are the front of the chest, side of the neck, and flexor aspects of the wrist (Fig. 1). The genital lesions are often said to occur chracteristically in a figure-eight pattern. However, this is not always the case, and in the lesion illustrated in Fig. 2, the perianal skin is not involved. Some authors recognizing the similarity between leukoplakia and lichen sclerosus et atrophicus believe that the two can be distinguished by the distribution of the lesions; thus, if the perineum and perianal areas are involved, the diagnosis is *ipso facto* lichen sclerosus et atrophicus; Taussig, on the contrary, described leukoplakic lesions in these areas. From the various descriptions there now seems little doubt that both macroscopically and microscopically the terms lichen sclerosus et atrophicus, atrophic leukoplakia, and kraurosis vulvae have been used to describe the same condition. In the interests of clarity, all these terms should be discarded. In 1961, Jeffcoate and Woodcock (11), recognizing that an accurate diagnosis could not be made from the gross appearance, proposed the use of a comprehensive term, chronic epithelial dystrophy.

VULVAL DYSTROPHY

A similar term—vulval dystrophy—was adopted by the International Society for the Study of Vulval Disease (ISSVD) in 1975 (9), and the older terms were discarded

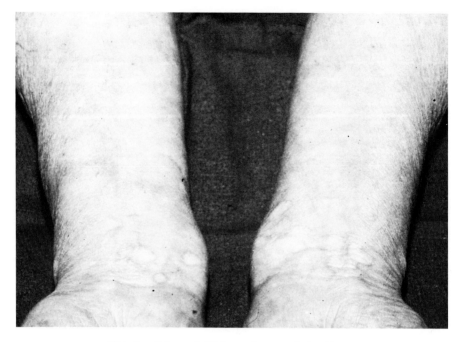

FIG. 1. Extragenital lichen sclerosus et atrophicus.

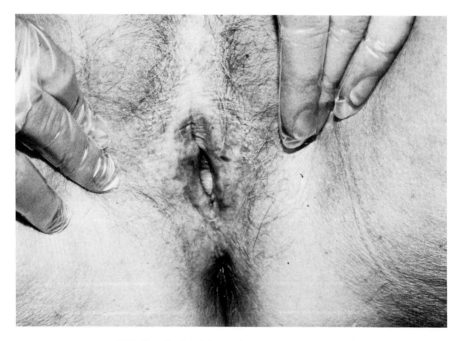

FIG. 2. Genital lichen sclerosus et atrophicus.

TABLE 4. *Recommendations of the ISSVD of terms to be discontinued (1975)*

Lichen sclerosus et atrophicus	Erythroplasia of Queyrat
Leukoplakia	Carcinoma simplex
Neurodermatitis	Leukoplakic vulvitis
Leukokeratosis	Hyperplastic vulvitis
Bowen's disease	Kraurosis vulvae

(Table 4). The new classification is shown in Table 5. Note that the term atrophicus has been omitted since the skin in this condition is now known to be metabolically active (4–5,17). All things considered, it would seem that the time has come again for a further modification of the ISSVD classification (Table 6). This involves four minor but significant changes:

1. In atrophic dystrophy (type II in Table 6), a subepithelial homogenous zone is not always to be found.

2. Since the homogeneous zone is said to be diagnostic of lichen sclerosus, although it has also been found by Taussig and others in atrophic leukoplakia, the term lichen sclerosus should be abandoned in favour of atrophic dystrophy.

3. It is recognized that atypic changes or even frank carcinoma may complicate the atrophic lesions characteristic of type II (Fig. 3).

4. Mixed dystrophy (type III) includes not only the association of atrophic and hypertrophic features in the same lesion but also the occurrence of atrophic and hypertrophic skin in adjacent areas.

SYMPTOMATOLOGY

The characteristic symptom of vulval dystrophy is itching, which varies in intensity and can be very severe. Dyspareunia may also accompany the pruritus but is seldom the presenting symptom and only rarely the sole feature. Occasionally, there is soreness and pain in the vulval area, and slight bleeding from excoriation and fissures can occur.

TABLE 5. *ISSVD classification (1975)*

I.	Hyperplastic dystrophy: hyperkeratosis, acanthosis, chronic inflammatory cell infiltrate a. without atypia b. with atypia
II.	Lichen sclerosus: hyperkeratosis, epithelial atrophy, subepithelial homogeneous zone, chronic inflammatory cell infiltrate
III.	Mixed dystrophy: hyperkeratosis, acanthosis, subepithelial homogeneous zone, chronic inflammatory cell infiltrate a. without atypia b. with atypia

TABLE 6.   *Proposed revised classification*

I.	Hypertrophic dystrophy: hyperkeratosis, acanthosis, chronic inflammatory cell infiltrate a. without atypia b. with atypia
II.	Atrophic dystrophy: hyperkeratosis, epidermal atrophy, ± subepithelial homogeneous zone, chronic inflammatory cell infiltrate a. without atypia b. with atypia
III.	Mixed dystrophy:[a] hyperkeratosis, acanthosis, subepithelial homogeneous zone, chronic inflammatory cell infiltrate a. without atypia b. with atypia

[a]Or adjacent areas of I and II.

RELATIONSHIP TO CARCINOMA

After the work of Berkeley and Bonney, and Taussig, leukoplakia was considered by many authors to be premalignant, which resulted in the widespread use of vulvectomy for such vulval lesions. However, in 1962, Jeffcoate (10) stated that although 5% of the patients with vulval dystrophy would have carcinoma in the initial biopsy, only an additional 5% would subsequently develop carcinoma, and all such patients would show atypia in the initial biopsy. Kaufman and Gardner (12) confirmed this in 1978 and estimated the incidence of carcinoma to be approximately 1 to 5%, always preceded by atypic changes.

In our experience, about 30% of patients had atypia, which was severe in none and moderate in only 8%. One patient had carcinoma *in situ*, which developed three years after mild atypia was diagnosed. The lesion was excised, and 10 years later the skin showed only mild atypia. Thus far, there has been no evidence of progression in any of the other patients.

AETIOLOGY

The aetiology of vulval dystrophy is unknown. Achlorhydria was noted in 1936 by Swift (14) as a related phenomenon, and Jeffcoate reported in 1962 (10) a 23% incidence of histamine-fast achlorhydria in his series of 269 patients with chronic vulval epithelial dystrophy. The 28 patients in our series were therefore offered a pentagastrin stimulation test to assess acid secretion, and 18 accepted. Of these, 10 had total achlorhydria, and the other 8 secreted acid normally.

There is general agreement that achlorhydria is an auto-immune phenomenon, and consequently evidence of other auto-immune conditions, such as the stigmata and/or signs of pernicious anaemia, hypothyroidism, and hyperthyroidism, was sought. Such evidence was found more often in this group of patients than in age-matched controls (Table 7).

Stomach hydrochloric acid secretion, an exocrine function, is regulated by the endocrine activity of gastrointestinal peptides, particularly gastrin (Fig. 4). This is

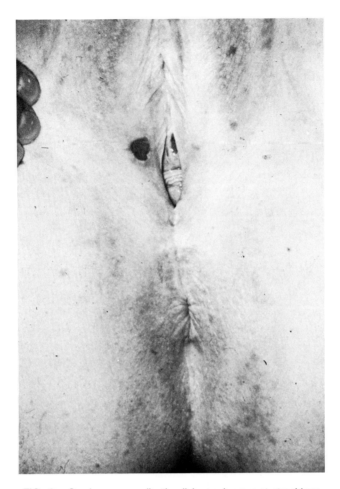

FIG. 3. Carcinoma complicating lichen sclerosus et atrophicus.

released from the G cells of the stomach and stimulates the parietal cells to produce hydrochloric acid, which by way of a feedback mechanism causes a decrease in gastrin production. Patients with achlorhydria would therefore be expected to have compensatory high circulating gastrin levels. Assays, however, produced results contrary to expectation, since only 3 patients had high gastrin levels, while 7 paradoxically had low levels (Table 8). To explain these low levels, three possibilities may be considered:

1. Laboratory error. This could be confidently excluded, since other samples examined on the same day gave the expected results.

2. The influence of other gastrin-depressing gastrointestinal peptides, especially vasoactive intestinal peptide (VIP) and somatostatin, which are known to reduce

TABLE 7. Summary of tests of significance (chi-square) comparing distributions of chronic vulval dystrophy patients with three selected groups of patients with respect to personal history of auto-immune disease and stigmata of pernicious anaemia as illustrated by seven clinical factors

Clinical factors	Case group[a] Chronic vulval dystrophy [1]	Auto-immune groups[a] Achlorhydria [2]	Pernicious anaemia [3]	Control group[a] Gynaecology in-patients [4]	Chi-square tests[b] Groups [1] vs [2]	Groups [1] vs [3]	Groups [1] vs [4]
Auto-immune disease							
Diabetes	2/26	8/25	4/25	2/25	S	NS	NS
Thyroid disease	7/26	5/25	8/25	2/25	NS	NS	T
Stigmata of pernicious anaemia							
Premature greying	7/26	5/25	5/25	0/25	NS	NS	HS
Raw tongue	7/26	8/25	17/25	2/25	NS	HS	T
Rhagades	6/26	7/25	7/25	0/25	NS	NS	S
Beefy tongue	1/26	3/25	1/25	0/25	NS	NS	NS
Blue eyes	10/26	13/25	14/25	15/25	NS	NS	NS

[a]Number of patients affected/total number in specified category.
[b]Chi-square tests were calculated by comparing group 1 with the three other groups separately.
NS: no significant difference between two selected levels at 5% ($p > 0.05$) level.
S: significant difference between two selected levels at 5% ($p = 0.05$) level.
HS: significant difference between two selected levels at 1% ($p = 0.01$) level.
T: significant difference between two selected levels at 10% ($p = 0.1$) level.

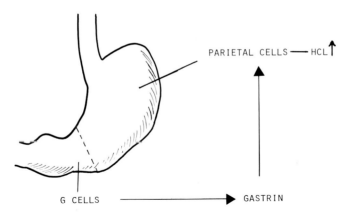

FIG. 4. Control of acid secretion. Relationship of gastrin to stomach hydrochloric-acid production. HCl: hydrochloric acid.

TABLE 8. *Correlation of plasma gastrin and stomach hydrochloric acid*

Hydrochloric acid	Plasma gastrin		
	Normal	High	Total
Normal	8	—	8
Absent	7	3	10

acid secretion. However, the plasma levels of these peptides were within normal limits in all 28 patients.

3. Deficient G cells.

a. Indirect evidence of associated auto-immune disease in these patients has already been shown by an abnormally high incidence of other auto-immune conditions. Direct evidence is currently being sought in blood assays of auto-antibodies to the G cells, the results of which are not yet available.

b. Hypoplasia. Gastric antral biopsies were performed, and no evidence of G-cell hypoplasia was found.

c. Chronic inflammation, however, was present in all. This, whether owing to auto-immune damage or not, could account for the paradoxically low gastrin level.

Pruritus is always associated with vulval dystrophy. Some gastrointestinal peptides not only lower gastrin and stomach acid but also serve as neurotransmitters, e.g., VIP, somatostatin, and substance P, all of which have been isolated from brain and neural tissue, the placenta, and the urogenital tract. All such peptides have been demonstrated in vulval skin *(unpublished data, 1980)*: substance P and somatostatin were always found, while VIP was found only occasionally. Somatostatin is of particular interest because of its high concentration in atrophic vulval dystrophies, where it may be implicated in the associated pruritus and achlorhydria, since it is not only a neurotransmitter but also inhibits gastrin and, indirectly, stomach-acid production.

In an effort to explain this occurrence of nonspecific vulval dystrophy, the following observations seem relevant:

1. Hypertrophic lesions can alter to atrophic and vice versa.
2. Achlorhydria is associated with both hypertrophic and atrophic lesions.
3. High somatostatin levels have been found in skin that has recently progressed from hypertrophic to atrophic dystrophy.
4. Decreasing levels of somatostatin have been observed in serial measurements from atrophic skin.
5. Atrophic skin, contrary to expected clinical appearances, is known to be metabolically active.
6. The association of vulval dystrophy and achlorhydria is not constant.

As a preliminary working hypothesis, it is therefore postulated that skin growth is under the control of a homeostatic feedback mechanism: increased cell growth is detected by a local control centre, which causes the release of an inhibiting substance, perhaps somatostatin, which leads to skin atrophy. This tends to cause decreased somatostatin production and skin hypertrophy. The net result is normal skin. To explain the association of vulval dystrophy and decreased acid secretion, it is suggested that in vulval dystrophy another gastrointestinal peptide, urogastrone, which is known to cause achlorhydria and increased epidermal cell growth (7), is abnormally elevated (Fig. 5). This results in hypertrophic vulval skin, which causes markedly increased levels of somatostatin. The resulting atrophy depresses somatostatin secretion, causing increased cell growth. Whereas in normal skin with normal urogastrone levels there is a balance between skin cell atrophy and hypertrophy, in vulval dystrophy the continuous stimulation engendered by abnormal levels of urogastrone leads to increased epidermal cell growth and consequently to

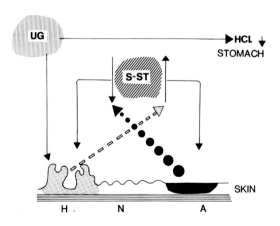

FIG. 5. Aetiology of chronic vulval dystrophy. UG: urogastrone; S-ST: somatostatin; H: hypertrophy; N: normal; A: atrophy; HCl: hydrochloric acid.

high rebound somatostatin levels. These cause decreased mitosis in the skin, which therefore alternates between hypertrophy and atrophy.

If the action of urogastrone on the vulval skin were unopposed, achlorhydria would be associated with only hypertrophic dystrophy. However, the local homeostatic mechanism in the vulva responds to the hypertrophy caused by urogastrone stimulation by releasing somatostatin locally, which causes atrophy. While the skin fluctuates between hypertrophy and atrophy, the gastric hydrochloric-acid secretion, under the unopposed influence of urogastrone, remains constantly depressed, since there is no rise in the plasma's somatostatin level.

Urogastrone stimulation causing hypertrophy results in extremely high rebound levels of somatostatin, which remain elevated in the skin even after atrophy has occurred. Consequently, high somatostatin levels persist for a time even in atrophic skin but eventually fall, as has been found in serial biopsies.

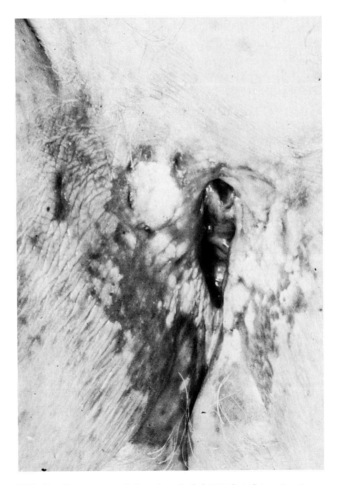

FIG. 6. Recurrence of chronic vulval dystrophy after vulvectomy.

The constant and opposing actions of urogastrone and somatostatin lead to hypertrophy and atrophy, respectively, continuously stimulating the skin cells; even atrophic skin has been shown to be metabolically active.

Finally, since much higher levels of urogastrone are required to cause achlorhydria than to cause epidermal cell growth, with lower levels of urogastrone vulval dystrophy may be present without achlorhydria.

TREATMENT

Initial biopsy is essential for accurate diagnosis and classification of vulval lesions. If carcinoma *in situ* or invasive carcinoma is found, a preliminary vulvectomy should be performed. Otherwise, there should be regular follow-up examinations at intervals of up to one year to monitor progress and permit repeat biopsy if necessary.

A search should be made for all possible aggravating features, such as candidiasis, trichomoniasis, allergies, or diabetes, and, if present, these should be energetically treated. Once the diagnosis has been made, the malignant potential evaluated, and all possible contributing factors eliminated, the treatment is primarily symptomatic and medical. Not only is vulvectomy a mutilating procedure but there is also a significant risk of recurrence of chronic vulval dystrophy (Fig. 6) and even carcinoma after such surgery (Fig. 7).

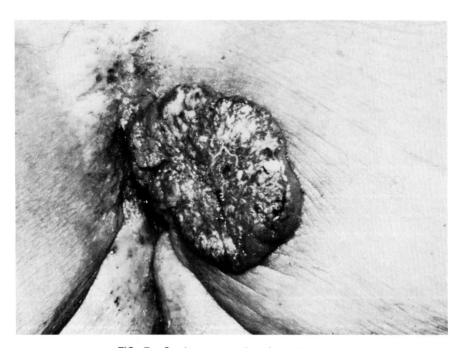

FIG. 7. Carcinoma occurring after vulvectomy.

Hyperplastic lesions usually do well with local corticosteroid creams. Hydrocortisone 0.5% is preferred to more potent preparations, such as the fluorinated compounds, since their prolonged use may lead to skin atrophy and vascular changes.

Atrophic lesions have in the past been treated similarly, although the logic is obviously dubious, since corticosteroid creams would be expected to cause further atrophy. Recently, testosterone ointment first suggested by Cinberg (3) in 1945, has been tried. It is said to thicken the skin and alleviate the symptoms. Rare side effects must be considered, including increased libido, clitoral enlargement, and facial hirsutism. The effects of local testosterone have been compared with the effects of a bland emollient using a double-blind technique. Vulval biopsy was performed initially and 6 weeks after the completion of each regimen. All patients with hypertrophic lesions exhibited a marked aggravation of the pruritus after testosterone, as did 6 of the 8 patients with atrophic lesions; the other 2 patients with atrophy of the vulval skin found that the pruritus was greatly relieved by testosterone. There were no histological skin changes in any patient.

SUMMARY

In describing vulval skin changes, all such terms as leukoplakia, kraurosis vulvae, and lichen sclerosus et atrophicus should be discarded in favour of chronic vulval dystrophy. Initial biopsy is mandatory to establish the precise diagnosis. From a review of the literature and from our own studies, we believe that vulval dystrophy is not usually a premalignant condition, a risk of carcinoma only existing in dystrophic vulvas with associated atypia. For such patients, the treatment is local vulvectomy; otherwise, the treatment should primarily be medical because of the high rate of recurrence of chronic vulval dystrophy after surgery. A working hypothesis of the aetiology of chronic vulval dysplasia is presented.

REFERENCES

1. Berkeley, C., and Bonney, V. (1909): Leukoplakic vulvitis and its relation to kraurosis vulvae and carcinoma vulvae. *Br. Med. J.*, 2:1739–1745.
2. Breisky, A. (1885): Über Kraurosis Vulvae. *Z. Heilk.*, 6:69–80.
3. Cinberg, B. L. (1945): Postmenopausal pruritus vulvae. *Am. J. Obstet. Gynecol.*, 49:647–657.
4. Clark, D. G. C., Zumoff, B., Brunschwig, A., and Hellman, L. (1960): Preferential uptake of phosphate by premalignant and malignant lesions of the vulva. *Cancer*, 13:775–779.
5. Friedrich, E. G., Julian, C. G., and Woodruff, G. D. (1964): Acridine organe fluorescence in vulval dysplasia. *Am. J. Obstet. Gynecol.*, 90:1281–1287.
6. Friedrich, E. G. (1976): Lichen sclerosus. *J. Reprod. Med.*, 17:147–163.
7. Gregory, H. (1980): Urogastrone: Isolation, structure, and basic functions. In: *Gastrointestinal Hormones*, edited by G. B. J. Glass, pp. 397–409. Raven Press, New York.
8. Hallopeau, H. (1887): Leçons clinique sur les maladies cutanées et syphilitiques. *Union Med.*, 43:742.
9. I.S.S.V.D. New nomenclature for vulval disease: 1 (1975): *Int. J. Gynaecol. Obstet.*, 13:237–239.
10. Jeffcoate, T. N. A. (1962): The dermatology of the vulva. *J. Obstet. Gynaecol. Br. Commonw.*, 69:888–890.
11. Jeffcoate, T. N. A., and Woodcock, A. S. (1961): Premalignant conditions of the vulva with particular reference to chronic epithelial dystrophies. *Br. Med. J.*, 2:127–134.

12. Kaufman, R. H., and Gardner, H. L. (1978): Vulval dystrophies. *Clin. Obstet. Gynecol.*, 21:1082–1106.
13. McAdams, A. J., and Kistner, R. W. (1958): The relationship of chronic vulval disease, leukoplakia and carcinoma in situ to carcinoma of the vulva. *Cancer*, 11:740–757.
14. Swift, B. H. (1936): Achlorhydria as an aetiological factor in pruritus vulvae associated with kraurosis in leukoplakia. *J. Obstet. Gynaecol. Br. Commonw.*, 43:1053–1077.
15. Taussig, F. J. (1929): Leukoplakic vulvitis and cancer of the vulva. *Am. J. Obstet. Gynecol.*, 18:472–503.
16. Wallace, H. J., and Whimster, I. W. (1951): Vulval atrophy and leukoplakia. *Br. J. Dermatol.*, 63:241–257.
17. Woodruff, J. D., Borkowf, H. I., Holzman, G. B., Arnold, E. A., and Knaack, J. (1965): Metabolic activity in normal and abnormal vulvar epithelia. *Am. J. Obstet. Gynecol.*, 91:809–819.

Recent Clinical Developments in Gynecologic Oncology, edited by C. Paul Morrow, et al.
Raven Press, New York © 1983.

Cryosurgery and "Cold" Coagulation in the Treatment of Cervical Intraepithelial Neoplasia

Ian D. Duncan

*Department of Obstetrics and Gynaecology, Ninewells Hospital and Medical School,
Dundee DD1 9SY, Scotland*

In areas where cervical cytology screening programmes have been carried out intensively, a reduction has been observed not only in the incidence of invasive squamous cervical cancer but in the mortality from such cancer as well (8). The Tayside Region in Scotland falls into this category (5), but as the number of patients with invasive squamous cervical carcinoma has declined, the number of patients identified with cervical intraepithelial neoplasia (CIN) has risen. The mean age at which the precursors of cervical cancer have been encountered has fallen, and in our own catchment area, the mean age of patients presenting with carcinoma *in situ* of the cervix has been consistently less than 35 years of age since 1972. Hysterectomy may be acceptable therapy to a patient whose family is complete and who suffers from persistent menorrhagia but is less acceptable to someone who wishes to have more children. In the latter case, cone biopsy is widely used, but even this treatment can adversely affect a patient's future childbearing ability (7).

The introduction of colposcopy has made it possible to significantly change the management of CIN. Diagnostic cone biopsy remains mandatory when the endocervical limit of a lesion cannot be seen or when there is any suspicion of invasive disease, which occurs in only a small proportion of patients. The expert colposcopist, with the skillful use of locally destructive techniques on the appropriate lesion in the appropriate patient, can reduce markedly the need for diagnostic and therapeutic cone biopsy.

PATIENTS AND METHODS

In 1975, a colposcopy clinic was established at Ninewells Hospital in Dundee, Scotland. Patients with abnormal cervical cytology are referred to the clinic, and at colposcopic examination directed punch biopsies are taken for histological diagnosis. Several different selective ablative techniques with different ranges of temperature have been evaluated, but most experience has been gained with cryo-surgery and, more recently, with "cold" coagulation at 100°C. Patients with biopsy-proven CIN are only considered for destruction of the lesion if the above criteria apply. Endocervical curettage is not carried out routinely, since it is felt that if the endocervical limit of the lesion can be seen, there is no question of any abnormality being present beyond this; moreover, as already stated, if the endocervical limit cannot be seen, cone biopsy is mandatory. Both ecto- and endocervical cytology employing a modified Ayre's spatula (4) are used for follow-up, and if an abnormal smear persists, then colposcopy is repeated and the patient dealt with as if she were a new referral.

Prior to October 1, 1980, 89 patients were treated with an M.T. 500 cryosurgical probe, employing nitrous oxide yielding a tip temperature of approximately −89°C. Thirty-six patients were treated with a single 5-min freeze, and 53 patients, with a double-freeze technique, consisting of two 3-min freezes separated by a 5-min thaw. The distribution of lesions is shown in Table 1.

After a 1975 pilot study, the Semm "cold" coagulator has been increasingly used at the clinic since April 1978, and 238 patients with CIN were treated on one occasion prior to October 1, 1980. The apparatus, as described by Semm (11), consists of a small, portable electronic monitor and a series of thermoprobes, the tip temperatures of which can be preselected. A temperature of 100°C was used throughout the study, and treatment areas were overlapped, with the different probes treating each area for 20 sec. Thus, the entire transformation zone and usually the lower endocervix were destroyed in approximately 100 sec. The distribution of lesions treated with the Semm coagulator is shown in Table 2.

Regardless of the mode of therapy, triple sulphonamide cream was prescribed for nightly application to the cervix for 1 week, but no sexual or sanitary restrictions were imposed. The mean age of the patients is shown in Table 3, with the ages ranging from 17 to 52 years.

RESULTS

The failure rates encountered with cryosurgery are shown in Table 4; all 8 failures were encountered within 18 months of treatment. The individual failures are de-

TABLE 1. *Distribution of cryosurgery patients*

		Freeze technique	
Grade	Lesion	Single	Double
CIN 3 (57)	CIS	7	35
	Severe dysplasia	4	11
CIN 2 (20)	Moderate dysplasia	18	2
CIN 1 (12)	Mild dysplasia	7	5
	Total	36	53

Numbers in parentheses indicate number of patients.
CIS: carcinoma *in situ.*

TABLE 2. *Distribution of "cold" coagulation patients*

Grade		Lesion	
CIN 3	(170)	CIS	(137)
		Severe dysplasia	(33)
CIN 2	(32)	Moderate dysplasia	
CIN 1	(36)	Mild dysplasia	
Total	238		

Numbers in parentheses indicate number of patients.
CIS: carcinoma *in situ.*

scribed in Table 5. All the patients had been treated with the double-freeze technique, and failures were encountered at all levels of abnormality. No cases of invasive cancer were encountered, and in only 1 patient was the subsequent lesion more severe than the original lesion. Further treatment of the patients was uniformly conservative.

The experience with "cold" coagulation has been more recent and follow-up accordingly shorter, but the failure rates are remarkably similar (Table 6). Again, all 13 failures discovered thus far have been within the first 18 months of follow-up. The treatment failures are described in Table 7, but particulars are incomplete in 1 patient, whose persistent abnormal cytology has as yet to be fully investigated. As with cryosurgery, failures occurred throughout the range of CIN. No invasive carcinomas developed, and in only 2 patients was the subsequent lesion more severe than the original lesion. "Cold" coagulation was repeated in 4 patients, apparently effectively in 2 and less certainly so in another 2.

SIDE EFFECTS AND COMPLICATIONS

Most patients experienced pelvic cramping lasting for the duration of the treatment, both with cryosurgery and "cold" coagulation. However, the discomfort disappeared almost immediately after treatment and was tolerated by all patients with no anaesthesia required.

TABLE 3. *Mean age of patients*

Lesion	Cryosurgery	"Cold" coagulation
CIS	28.0 ± 4.2 yr	29.5 ± 6.0 yr
Severe dysplasia	27.5 ± 7.0	29.7 ± 5.2
Moderate dysplasia	28.6 ± 5.2	28.3 ± 5.6
Mild dysplasia	28.8 ± 6.8	30.9 ± 8.0
All CIN	28.1 ± 5.3	29.6 ± 6.2

CIS: carcinoma *in situ.*

TABLE 4. *Failure rates with cryosurgery*

			Duration of follow-up			
Lesion	1st six months[a]	2nd six months[a]	3rd six months[a]	4th six months[a]	5th six months[a]	6th six months[a]
Carcinoma in situ	3/42 = 7%	1/37 = 2.5%	0/32 = Nil	0/28 = Nil	0/19 = Nil	0/9 = Nil
SD	1/15 = 6.5%	0/14 = Nil	1/14 = 7%	0/13 = Nil	0/11 = Nil	0/6 = Nil
CIN 2	1/20 = 5%	0/17 = Nil	0/15 = Nil	0/15 = Nil	0/8 = Nil	0/3 = Nil
CIN 1	0/12 = Nil	0/11 = Nil	1/11 = 9%	0/6 = Nil	0/4 = Nil	0/2 = Nil
All CIN	5/89 = 5.5%	1/79 = 1.5%	2/72 = 3%	0/62 = Nil	0/42 = Nil	0/20 = Nil

[a]Number of failures/total number of patients.
CIS: carcinoma *in situ*; SD: severe dysplasia.

TABLE 5. *Treatment failure with cryosurgery*

Patient	Age[a]	Original lesion	Freeze	Subsequent lesion	Further treatment	Current cytology
M.A.	34	CIS	Double	SD	"Cold" coag.	Normal
M.M.	27	CIS	Double	CIN 1	"Cold" coag.	Normal
				CIS	Cone biopsy	
M.R.	35	CIS	Double	CIN 1	Punch biopsy	Normal
M.S.	30	CIS	Double	CIN 1	Cone biopsy	Normal
E.B.	41	SD	Double	SD	"Cold" coag.	Normal
B.N.	21	SD	Double	CIN 1	Punch biopsy	Normal
J.A.	24	CIN 2	Double	CIS	"Cold" coag.	Normal
				CIS	"Cold" coag.	
L.W.	25	CIN 1	Double	CIN 1	Punch biopsy	Normal

[a]Mean age: 29.6 ± 6.2 yr.
CIS: carcinoma *in situ;* SD: severe dysplasia.

Patients were forewarned that they might experience some vaginal discharge; this was not the case with patients treated with "cold" coagulation but was frequently encountered by patients treated with cryosurgery. Secondary haemorrhage occurred in less than 2% of the patients in both groups and was always minor, requiring no hospitalisation or special treatment. One patient treated with "cold" coagulation developed symptoms suggestive of pelvic inflammatory disease, but they disappeared with the administration of metronidazole. One patient with irregular periods was inadvertently treated at 5 weeks' gestation with the "cold" coagulator, and she aborted one week later.

SUBSEQUENT PREGNANCY

A close record was kept during follow-up of the patients' contraceptive practices and marital status; fertility after treatment with cryosurgery and "cold" coagulation is demonstrated in Tables 8 and 9, respectively. Impairment of fertility was not obviously encountered. Operative intervention was rarely called for, and most

TABLE 6. *Failure rates with "cold" coagulation*

Lesion	Duration of follow-up				
	1st six months[a]	2nd six months[a]	3rd six months[a]	4th six months[a]	5th six months[a]
CIS	5/137 = 3.5%	3/82 = 3.5%	1/45 = 2%	0/27 = Nil	0/6 = Nil
SD	0/33 = Nil	0/15 = Nil	0/5 = Nil	0/3 = Nil	
CIN 2	1/32 = 3%	2/15 = 13.5%	0/6 = Nil	0/2 = Nil	
CIN 1	1/36 = 3%	0/20 = Nil	0/12 = Nil	0/7 = Nil	0/2 = Nil
All CIN	7/238 = 3%	5/132 = 4%	1/86 = 1.5%	0/39 = Nil	0/8 = Nil

[a]Number of failures/total no. of patients.
CIS: carcinoma *in situ;* SD: severe dysplasia.

TABLE 7. *Treatment failures with "cold" coagulation*

Patient	Age[a]	Original lesion	Subsequent lesion	Further treatment	Current cytology
M.B.	30	CIS	CIS	Cone biopsy hysterectomy	Normal
P.N.	34	CIS	CIS	Hysterectomy	Normal
J.C.	28	CIS	CIS	"Cold" coagulation	Class 2
J.A.	25	CIS	CIS	"Cold" coagulation	Class 2
J.C.	27	CIS	SD	"Cold" coagulation	Normal
M.S.	40	CIS	SD	Hysterectomy	Normal
C.McR.	25	CIS	CIN 2	Hysterectomy	Normal
C.C.	32	CIS	CIN 1	Hysterectomy	Normal
M.R.	30	CIS	CIN 1	"Cold" coagulation	Normal
M.C.	28	CIN 2	CIS	Hysterectomy	Normal
P.McD.	30	CIN 2	CIN 2	Nil	Class 3
J.M.	25	CIN 2			Class 3
M.M.	27	CIN 1	CIS	Cone biopsy	Normal

[a]Mean age: 29.3 ± 4.2 yr.
CIS: carcinoma *in situ;* SD: severe dysplasia.

pregnancies progressed to spontaneous delivery at term. Cervical cerclage was avoided, except in 1 patient treated with "cold" coagulation for CIN 3 persisting after cone biopsy. Therapeutically aborted pregnancies reflect the social circumstances of each patient. As a comparison, 18% of the 89 patients treated with cryosurgery and 15.5% of the 238 patients treated with "cold" coagulation had had a therapeutic abortion prior to treatment.

DISCUSSION

Regardless of the type of selective ablation used, the technique must be capable of destroying both the surface epithelium and the abnormal epithelium within the cervical crypts. Przybora and Plutowa (10) described 56 cases of carcinoma *in situ*

TABLE 8. *Fertility after cryosurgery*

	No.	Fertility
	2	Preexisting infertility
	1	No conception after six months
	15	Spontaneous delivery at term
24[a]	1	Spontaneous delivery at 35 weeks
	1	Forceps delivery at term
	3	Currently pregnant
	1	Spontaneous first trimester abortion
	2	Therapeutic abortion
		Conception rate 19/20 = 95%

[a]Only 20 patients are actually involved here, since 4 of the patients had 2 pregnancies.

TABLE 9. *Fertility after "cold" coagulation*

No.	Fertility
6	Prexisting infertility (3 to 15 yr)
1	No conception after 10 months
21	Spontaneous delivery at term
2	Lower uterine segment Caesarean section
	1 twin breeches
	1 fetal distress
2	Left area pregnant
1	Currently pregnant
2	Missed abortions at 16 weeks
7	Therapeutic abortion

36 {

Conception rate 35/36 = 97.2%

in which there was significant crypt involvement, and in no case was this more than 4 mm deep. In 52 cases, it was less than 3 mm. Anderson and Hartley (1) found the mean depth of crypt involvement with CIN 3 to be 1.24 mm in 343 therapeutic cone biopsies. In 95% of their patients, crypt involvement did not exceed 2.91 mm and in 99.7%, it was 3.8 mm or less. This gives an indication of the necessary depth of destruction.

Of the various methods used, cryosurgery has probably been used the most extensively. The subject was recently reviewed by Charles and Savage (3), who reported cure rates as low as 27.3% and as high as 96%. Ostergard (9) recently cautioned that in his experience there were more treatment failures in patients with carcinoma *in situ* than in patients with lesser degrees of abnormality; however, only 18 patients (of whom 7 experienced failure) could be adequately assessed. Cryosurgery has been criticised because it results in scarring of the transformation zone and retraction of the neosquamocolumnar junction, thus rendering colposcopic follow-up unsatisfactory. Chanen (2), however, argues that this end result, which he achieves by electrocautery, is desirable, since the cervical portio becomes completely covered with mature stable squamous epithelium with no malignant potential. As described above, we employ routine ecto- and endocervical scrapes to ensure adequate posttreatment cytological assessment of both zones.

When a cryosurgical apparatus with a small gas reservoir is used repeatedly, it can "freeze up," requiring a change of gas cylinder, which in a busy colposcopy clinic takes up needed time. In addition, copious vaginal discharge is usually experienced by the patient. However, Fergusson and Craft (6) reported less posttreatment discharge with the use of the Semm "cold" coagulator in the treatment of benign cervical "erosion." This led to the introduction and investigation of the "cold" coagulator in the treatment of CIN at the Ninewells Colposcopy Clinic. The results obtained thus far indicate that it is effective and essentially free from side effects and that it does not impair subsequent fertility. It is well tolerated by patients and is unaccompanied by smoke, smell, or noise. The sensation experienced by the patient is similar to that experienced with other forms of selective ablation but is of very short duration. The capital and running costs are low. Our experience is shared by Staland (13), who in 1978 reported only 2 cases of persistence of suspicious cytology in 71 patients with premalignant lesions of the uterine cervix treated with the Semm "cold" coagulator. Of course, it is clear that long-term follow-up is necessary, and it is currently being carried out in our unit.

If strict criteria are not adhered to, tragedy can result (12). However, given the right lesion in the right patient after accurate colposcopic and histological assessment, such simple procedures as cryosurgery and "cold" coagulation can return the premalignant cervix to normal, permitting further childbearing and reducing the need for cone biopsy or hysterectomy.

REFERENCES

1. Anderson, M. C., and Hartley, R. B. (1980): Cervical crypt involvement by intraepithelial neoplasia. *Obstet. Gynecol.*, 55:546–550.
2. Chanen, W. (1981): Radical electrocoagulation diathermy. In: *Gynecologic Oncology: Fundamental Principles and Clinical Practice*, edited by M. Coppleson, pp. 815–821. Churchill Livingstone, London.
3. Charles, E. H., and Savage, E. W. (1980): Cryosurgical treatment of cervical intraepithelial neoplasia. *Obstet. Gynecol. Surv.*, 35:539–548.
4. Duguid, H. L. D., Parratt, D., and Traynor, R. (1980): Actinomyces-like organisms in cervical smears from women using intra-uterine contraceptive devices. *Br. Med. J.*, 281:534–537.
5. Duncan, I. D. (1981): Management of Stage I Carcinoma of Cervix. In: *Progress in Obstetrics and Gynaecology, Vol. 1*, edited by J. Studd, pp. 217–228. Churchill Livingstone, London.
6. Fergusson, I. L. C., and Craft, J. L. (1974): A new "Cold Coagulator" for use in the out-patient treatment of cervical erosion. *J. Obstet. Gynaecol. Br. Commonw.*, 81:324–327.
7. Jones, J. M., and Sweetnam, P. M. (1982): Cardiff cervical cytology study. Morbidity from and effectiveness of cone biopsy of cervix. In: *Proceedings of Fourth World Congress*, edited by M. C. Anderson, pp. 99–102. International Federation for Cervical Pathology and Colposcopy, London.
8. Macgregor, J. E., and Teper, S. (1978): Mortality from carcinoma of cervix uteri in Britain. *Lancet*, 2:774–776.
9. Ostergard, D. R. (1980): Cryosurgical treatment of cervical intraepithelial neoplasia. *Obstet. Gynecol.*, 56:231–233.
10. Przybora, L. A., and Plutowa, A. (1959): Histological topography of carcinoma in situ of the cervix uteri. *Cancer*, 12:263–277.
11. Semm, K. (1966): New apparatus for the "Cold-Coagulation" of benign cervical lesions. *Am. J. Obstet. Gynecol.*, 95:963–966.
12. Sevin, B. U., Ford, J. H., Girtanner, R. D., Hoskins, W. J., Ng, A. B. P., Nordqvist, S. R. B., and Averette, H. E. (1979): Invasive cancer of the cervix after cryosurgery. Pitfalls of conservative management. *Obstet. Gynecol.*, 53:465–471.
13. Staland, B. (1978): Treatment of premalignant lesions of the uterine cervix by means of moderate heat thermo-surgery using the Semm coagulator. *Ann. Chir. Gynaecol.*, 67:112–116.

Recent Clinical Developments in Gynecologic Oncology, edited by C. Paul Morrow, et al. Raven Press, New York © 1983.

Nuclear and Cytoplasmic Oestrogen Receptors in Squamous Carcinoma of the Cervix

*W. P. Soutter[1], **R. J. Pegoraro, *R. W. Green-Thompson, *D. V. Naidoo, **S. M. Joubert, and *R. H. Philpott

*Department of Gynaecology and **Department of Chemical Pathology, Faculty of Medicine, University of Natal, Durban, Republic of South Africa

The human uterine cervix is an oestrogen-responsive organ: the cervical stroma grows under the influence of oestrogens at puberty, during pregnancy, and when oral contraceptives are used; the columnar epithelium of the endocervix secretes mucus in response to oestrogens; and the squamous epithelium of the ectocervix grows in response to oestrogens, as can be seen when the atrophic cervix of a postmenopausal woman is treated with oestrogens. Invasive squamous carcinoma of the cervix develops from abnormal squamous metaplasia in the transformation zone, which results from oestrogen-promoted hypertrophy and eversion of the cervix.

There is now considerable evidence in animals (1,2,17) and humans (4,15) that oestrogens produce their effects by interacting with intracellular receptors and that the nuclear-bound receptors are of particular importance in this respect. An intact oestrogen-receptor mechanism in breast cancer implies an improved prognosis (12) and a high probability of response to endocrine therapy (13). The study discussed in this chapter was undertaken to determine whether or not cytoplasmic and nuclear oestrogen receptors are present in squamous cervical cancer.

MATERIALS AND METHODS

The uteri from eight women undergoing hysterectomy because of fibroids were obtained immediately after removal. Endometrium was scraped out of the uterine cavity, and endocervical, ectocervical, and stromal tissues were dissected from the cervix, placed in buffered saline (BS; 0.15 mole/litre NaCl, 20 mmole/litre Hepes,

---

[1]*Present address:* Department of Obstetrics and Gynaecology, University of Sheffield, The Jessop Hospital for Women, Sheffield S3 7RE, England

pH 7.4) on ice, and transported to the laboratory for immediate assay. The uterus was sent for routine histological examination to confirm the normality of the tissues obtained.

Biopsies were obtained from the tumours of 58 women with squamous carcinoma of the cervix. One portion was placed in formol saline for histological confirmation of the diagnosis. The remainder was transported immediately to the laboratory in BS on ice and was either assayed immediately or stored in liquid nitrogen for not more than four weeks.

$(2,4,6,7-^3H)$-Oestradiol-17β (85 to 110 Ci/mmole) was obtained from the Radiochemical Centre, Amersham, England, and its purity was confirmed by ascending paper chromatography (6). Unlabelled steroids were obtained from the Sigma Co. (St. Louis, Missouri), and, unless otherwise stated, all other chemicals were obtained from E. Merck (Darmstadt, Germany). The assay has been described in detail previously (23,18) and therefore will be outlined only briefly here to indicate modifications in technique. Normal stroma and squamous epithelium were more readily homogenised using a microdismembrator (Braun, Melsunge, West Germany), but the less fibrous tissues from the endometrium and the endocervix and most tumour samples were disrupted using a Teflon-glass homogeniser. The following homogenising buffer (HED) was used: 20 mmole/litre Hepes, 1.5 mmole/litre ethylenediametetraacetate (EDTA), 0.25 mmole/litre dithiothreitol, pH 7.4. Only 150 mg tissue (50 mg/ml HED) were required for a full assay. A crude nuclear pellet was prepared by centrifugation at 700 g for 10 min, the supernatant was decanted, and a portion was stored at $-20°C$ for protein estimation (14). The crude nuclear pellet was washed once in BS and then resuspended in 0.15 mmole/litre NaCl, 20 mmole/litre Hepes, pH 6.2 and an aliquot kept at $-20°C$ for DNA estimation (10). The binding of (^3H)-oestradiol-17β in both the 700 g supernatant (cytoplasmic binding) and the resuspended nuclear pellet was measured in eight 150-μl portions after incubation for 18 hr at 4°C with (^3H)-oestradiol-17β at final concentrations of 0.1 to 0.8 nmole/litre. An additional portion from both fractions was incubated with 0.8 nmole/litre (^3H)-oestradiol-17β and a hundredfold excess of nonradioactive diethylstilboestrol to measure nonspecific binding. Appropriate blanks were included in the cytoplasmic assay. Free and loosely bound ligand was removed from the cytoplasmic preparation by dextran-coated charcoal; from the nuclear suspension it was removed by washing with 20 ml 0.15 mole/litre NaCl on Whatman GF/C filters using a millipore filter unit. Total radioactivity and bound radioactivity were measured in a Packard Tricarb 3390 using Instagel (Packard) as the scintillant at average efficiencies of 26% for the cytoplasmic assay and 42% for the nuclear assay. The data were plotted according to Scatchard (21), and a straight line was drawn by the method of least squares using the linear part of the plot. The correlation coefficient of the line so drawn was required to be significant at least at the 5% level. The number of binding sites was calculated from the point of interception of this line and the abscissa, and the dissociation constant, which is inversely proportional to the strength of the binding measured, was calculated from the reciprocal of the slope. Receptors were deemed to be present if the dissociation constant was less than 8×10^{-10} mole/litre. Thus, it was possible in every case to measure the number of receptors present and the strength of the binding.

TABLE 1. *Means and ranges of oestrogen receptor results in normal uterine tissue*

		CER			NER	
Uterine tissue	N	fmol E$_2$/mg protein	K$_D$ × 10^{-10} mol/litre	N	fmol E$_2$/mg DNA	K$_D$ × 10^{-10} mol /litre
Endometrium	8	173 (35–324)	0.82 (0.35–1.33)	7[a]	337 (189–2,091)	1.56 (0.30–4.34)
Endocervix	8	91 (36–235)	1.00 (0.49–3.72)	7[a]	512 (200–921)	2.21 (0.59–5.39)
Ectocervix	8	83 (39–329)	2.32 (0.96–4.68)	7[a]	645 (459–984)	3.00 (1.04–6.91)
Stroma	8	57 (23–125)	2.67 (0.87–7.81)	7[a]	1,157 (514–1,785)	2.64 (0.5–5.24)

[a]One assay from this group was technically unsatisfactory.
Numbers in parentheses indicate ranges.

RESULTS

All three components of the 8 normal cervices examined contained both nuclear receptors (NER) and cytoplasmic receptors (CER) (Table 1). Although there seemed to be lower concentrations of CER in the cervical tissues than in the endometrium, no such difference was apparent for NER.

By contrast, samples of squamous carcinoma contained both CER and NER in 19% of the cases, CER alone in 52% of the cases, and NER alone in two specimens (Table 2). The levels of receptor concentrations found were lower than in normal cervical tissue (Table 3). Examples of Scatchard plots of the data are shown in Figs. 1 to 3. There was no correlation between CER and NER concentrations in tumours with receptor present (Fig. 4).

The records of the first 40 patients studied were examined for data on the age and menopausal status of the subjects. In 6 cases, the age had not been recorded, either because it was not known or because it could not be determined accurately. In another 3 patients (aged 37, 39, and 43 years), the menopausal status had been omitted from the records. It seemed that tumours with neither CER nor NER were more common in younger, premenopausal women (Tables 4 and 5).

TABLE 2. *Oestrogen receptors in squamous carcinoma of the cervix*

CER/NER	N	%
+/+	11	19
+/−	30	52
−/+	2	3
−/−	15	26
Total	58	100

TABLE 3. *Oestrogen receptor levels and dissociation constants in squamous carcinoma of the cervix*

	CER		NER	
	fmole E_2/mg protein	$K_D \times 10^{-10}$ mole/litre	fmole E_2/mg DNA	$K_D \times 10^{-10}$ mole/litre
Mean	28	2.59	187	2.87
SEM	2.78	0.26	23.7	0.20
Range	5–96	0.34–6.84	61–397	1.53–4.47
Number	41	41	13	13

DISCUSSION

The limited study of normal cervical tissues reported in this chapter was intended only to demonstrate that oestrogen receptors are normally present in the nucleus of the cells as well as in the cytoplasm. The cytoplasmic levels found are similar to those demonstrated by Sanborn and co-workers (20).

In earlier studies of carcinoma of the cervix, a smaller proportion of tumours was found to show evidence of oestrogen binding. Whole tissue uptake studies

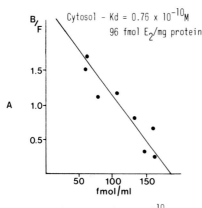

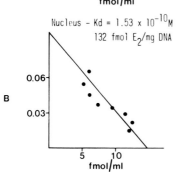

FIG. 1. Scatchard plots of data from squamous carcinoma of cervix showing both CER **(A)** and NER **(B)**. (From Soutter et al. (24), with permission.)

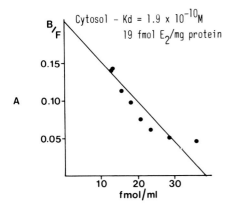

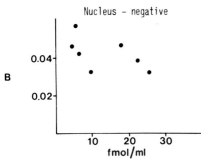

FIG. 2. Scatchard plots of data from squamous carcinoma of cervix showing CER **(A)** but no NER **(B)**. (From Soutter et al. (24), with permission.)

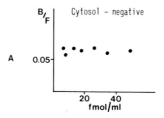

FIG. 3. Scatchard plots of data from squamous carcinoma of cervix showing no CER **(A)** but NER **(B)**. (From Soutter et al. (24), with permission.)

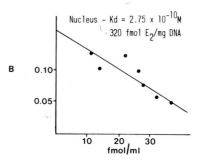

TABLE 4. *Age and oestrogen receptor status*

	CER/NER				
Age (yr)	+/+	+/−	−/+	−/−	Total
<45	2	12	0	6	20
>45	3	9	2	0	14
Total	5	21	2	6	34

TABLE 5. *Menopausal and receptor status*

	CER/NER				
	+/+	+/−	−/+	−/−	Total
Premenopausal	1	9	0	5	15
Postmenopausal	3	10	2	1	16
Total	4	19	2	6	31

showed low levels of binding in 10 of 26 samples (27). Cytoplasmic receptor measurement gave positive results at very low levels of binding in 17% of 42 samples of squamous carcinoma but in 3 of 4 samples of adenocarcinoma of the cervix (8). However, in a study of several tissues and tumours, the 3 samples of carcinoma of the cervix that were assayed were all found to contain cytoplasmic oestrogen receptors (26).

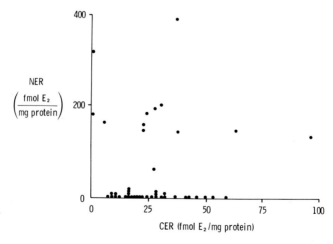

FIG. 4. Plot of CER against NER in squamous cervical carcinomas containing oestrogen receptors.

Since the assay used in this study was able to detect receptors in normal tissue, it may have been possible that the low levels of receptors found in the tumours were caused by an admixture of normal cells in the biopsy specimen. A histological assessment of this "contamination" showed that in the majority of cases, the amount of normal tissue present was too small to account for the concentrations of receptor detected, and there was no relation between the percentage of tumour cells in the biopsy and the results of the receptor assay (24). Thus it seems unlikely that the receptors detected in biopsies of tumour tissue were present only in normal cells contained in the sample.

Studies on the effect of age and menopausal status on the CER content of breast cancers generally have indicated a lower percentage of CER-positive tumours in premenopausal women than in postmenopausal women and higher CER concentrations with increasing age (3,16). This has been explained in two ways. In the first explanation it was thought that CER occupied by endogenous oestradiol would not be measurable by current assays. This argument is untenable, since CER-negative tumours contain lower concentrations of oestradiol than CER-positive samples, and there is no correlation between CER levels and the amount of oestradiol in CER-positive tumours (7). The second explanation was that CER would be translocated to the nucleus by the higher endogenous oestradiol levels found in premenopausal women. However, using an assay that is almost identical to the one described in this chapter and that has been shown to measure receptors occupied by endogenous oestradiol (22), Leake and co-workers (11) found higher concentrations of both CER and NER in breast cancers from postmenopausal patients than from premenopausal patients. It therefore seems likely that the higher incidence of CER- and NER-negative cervical cancers seen in younger, premenopausal women in this study reflects a characteristic of the tumour itself rather than of the tumour's hormonal environment. This feature may be relevant with respect to the appropriate therapy and the prognosis.

Tumours containing both CER and NER may be susceptible to oestrogen regulation. Seventy-one percent of breast cancers with this receptor configuration respond to endocrine therapy (13). It may also be significant that the probability of a response to endocrine therapy is not related to the absolute value of CER measured (4). Tumours with cytoplasmic but no nuclear binding may have abnormal receptors that are incapable of translocation to the nucleus. Such tumours are much less common in breast cancer, where they account for 12 to 17% of cases (13,18), of which a surprisingly high 24% respond to endocrine therapy (13). Tumours with receptors, found only in the nucleus remain an enigma in both breast (13) and cervical carcinoma and challenge current concepts of oestrogen action. Few breast tumours of this type respond to endocrine therapy (13). Similarly, by extrapolation from breast-cancer experience, few tumours with no evidence of oestrogen receptors in either compartment would be expected to respond to endocrine therapy (13) and may be expected to carry a poorer prognosis (12).

It would be quite erroneous to draw conclusions from experience with breast cancer about the outcome of endocrine therapy or the prognosis in carcinoma of the cervix simply because some of both types of cancer contain oestrogen receptors.

The concentrations of both CER and NER are somewhat lower in carcinoma of the cervix than in carcinoma of the breast (13,18), although the lack of correlation between CER levels and the response to endocrine therapy has already been mentioned; however, other, more subtle, differences may exist. There is evidence that endocrine therapy in recurrent carcinoma of the cervix will produce a response in about 27% of cases, a figure similar to the response rate in breast cancer, a tumor widely considered to be hormone responsive (5). Furthermore, it is most encouraging to note that 2 controlled studies of oestrogen therapy combined with radiotherapy as the primary treatment of carcinoma of the cervix have shown a clear and substantial improvement in the 5-year survival rate of patients given oestrogens (19,25). If the mode of action of oestrogens in carcinoma of the cervix is similar to that in carcinoma of the breast, antioestrogens may be equally effective (9) and the measurement of progesterone receptors valuable (3).

ACKNOWLEDGMENT

This study was supported by the South African Medical Research Council through the Preclinical Diagnostic Chemistry Research Group.

REFERENCES

1. Anderson, J. N., Peck, E. J., and Clark, J. H. (1974): Nuclear receptor oestradiol complex: a requirement for uterotrophic responses. *Endocrinology*, 95:174–178.
2. Anderson, J. N., Peck, E. J., and Clark, J. H. (1975): Oestrogen-induced uterine responses and growth: relationship to receptor oestrogen binding by uterine nuclei. *Endocrinology*, 96:160–167.
3. Barnes, D. M., Skinner, L. G., and Ribeiro, G. G. (1979): Triple hormone receptor assay: a more accurate predictive tool for the treatment of advanced breast cancer? *Br. J. Cancer*, 40:862–865.
4. Barnes, D. M., Ribeiro, G. G., and Skinner, L. G. (1979): Simultaneous estimation of oestrogen and progestin receptor activity in human breast tumours and correlation with response to treatment. In: *Steroid Receptor Assays in Human Breast Tumours*, edited by R. J. B. King, pp. 16–32. Alpha Omega Publishing, Cardiff.
5. Briggs, M. H., Caldwell, A. D. S., and Pitchford, A. G. (1967): Sex hormones in female cancer. *Lancet*, 2:100.
6. Bush, I. E. (1952): Methods of paper chromatography of steroids applicable to the study of steroids in mammalian blood and tissues. *Biochem. J.*, 50:370–378.
7. Edery, M., Goussard, J., Dehennin, L., Scholler, R., Reiffsteck, J., and Drosdowsky, M. A. (1981): Endogenous oestradiol-17β concentration in breast tumours determined by mass fragmentography and by radioimmunoassay: relationship to receptor content. *Eur. J. Cancer*, 17:115–120.
8. Hähnel, R., Martin, J. D., Masters, A. M., Ratajezak, T., and Twaddle, E. (1979): Oestrogen receptors and blood hormone levels in cervical carcinoma and other gynaecological tumours. *Gynecol. Oncol.*, 8:226–233.
9. Ingle, J. N., Ahmann, D. L., Green, S. J., Edmonson, J. H., Bisel, H. F., Kvols, L. K., Nichols, W. C., Creagan, E. T., Hahn, R. G., Rubin, J., and Frytak, S. (1981): Randomized clinical trial of diethylstilboestrol versus tamoxifen in post-menopausal women with advanced breast cancer. *N. Engl. J. Med.*, 304:16–21.
10. Katzenellenbogen, B. S., and Leake, R. E. (1974): Distribution of the oestrogen-induced protein and of total protein between endometrial and myometrial fractions of the immature and mature rat uterus. *J. Endocrinol.*, 63:439–449.
11. Leake, R. E., Laing, L., and Smith, D. C. (1979): A role for nuclear oestrogen receptors in prediction of therapy regime for breast cancer patients. In: *Steroid Receptor Assays in Human Breast Tumours*, edited by R. J. B. King, pp. 73–85. Alpha Omega Publishing, Cardiff.

12. Leake, R. E., Laing, L., McArdle, C., and Smith, D. C. (1981): Soluble and nuclear oestrogen receptor status in human breast cancer in relation to prognosis. *Br. J. Cancer*, 43:67–71.
13. Leake, R. E., Laing, L., Calman, K. C., Macbeth, F. R., Crawford, D., and Smith, D. C. (1981): Oestrogen receptor status and endocrine therapy of breast cancer: response rate and status stability. *Br. J. Cancer*, 43:59–66.
14. Lowry, O. H., Rosenbrough, N. J., Farr, A. L., and Randall, R. J. (1951): Protein measurement with the Folin phenol reagent. *J. Biol. Chem.*, 193:265–275.
15. McGuire, W. L., Zava, D. T., Horwitz, K. B., Garola, R. E., and Chamness, G. C. (1978): Receptors and breast cancer: do we know it all? *J. Steroid Biochem.*, 9:461–466.
16. Maynard, P. V., and Griffiths, K. (1979): Clinical, pathological and biochemical aspects of the oestrogen receptor in primary human breast cancer. In: *Steroid Receptor Assays in Human Breast Tumours*, edited by R. J. B. King, pp. 86–99. Alpha Omega Publishing, Cardiff.
17. O'Malley, B. W., and Means, A. R. (1974): Female steroid hormones and target cell nuclei. *Science*, 183:610–620.
18. Pegoraro, R. J., Soutter, W. P., Joubert, S. M., Nirmul, D., and Bryer, J. V. (1980): Nuclear and cytoplasmic oestrogen receptors in human mammary carcinoma. *S. Afr. Med. J.*, 58:807–813.
19. Runge, H. (1959): Zusätzliche Hormonbehandlung des Krebses. *Arch. Gynaek.*, 193:122–138.
20. Sanborn, B. M., Kuo, H. S., and Held, B. (1978): Oestrogen and progesterone binding site concentrations in human endometrium and cervix throughout the menstrual cycle and in tissue from women taking oral contraceptives. *J. Steroid Biochem.*, 9:951–955.
21. Scatchard, G. (1949): The attraction of proteins for small molecules and ions. *Ann. N.Y. Acad. Sci.*, 51:660–672.
22. Soutter, W. P. (1979): Oestrogen uptake and high affinity binding, and RNA polymerase activity in normal and abnormal human endometrium. *M.D. Thesis*, University of Glasgow.
23. Soutter, W. P., Hamilton, K., and Leake, R. E. (1979): High affinity binding of oestradiol-17β in the nuclei of human endometrial cells. *J. Steroid Biochem.*, 10:529–534.
24. Soutter, W. P., Pegoraro, R. J., Green-Thompson, R. W., Naidoo, D. V., Joubert, S. M., Philpott, R. H. (1981): Nuclear and cytoplasmic oestrogen receptors in squamous carcinoma of the cervix. *Br. J. Cancer*, 44:154–159.
25. Sugimori, M., Taki, I., and Koga, K. (1976): Adjuvant hormone therapy to radiation treatment for cervical cancer. *Acta Obstet. Gynaecol. Jpn.*, 23:77–82.
26. Syrjälä, P., Kontula, K., Jänne, O., Kauppila, A., and Vihko, R. (1978): Steroid receptors in normal and neoplastic human uterine tissue. In: *Endometrial Cancer*, edited by M. G. Brush, R. J. B. King, and R. W. Taylor, pp. 242–251. Balliere Tindall, London.
27. Terenius, L., Lindell, A., and Persson, B. H. (1971): Binding of oestradiol-17β to human cancer tissue of the female genital tract. *Cancer Res.*, 31:1895–1898.

Recent Clinical Developments in Gynecologic Oncology, edited by C. Paul Morrow, et al. Raven Press, New York © 1983.

Value and Complications of Periaortic Irradiation in Advanced Cervical Cancer

Per Kolstad

Department of Gynecology, The Norwegian Radium Hospital, Oslo 3, Norway

Treatment with radiotherapy dates to the beginning of the 20th century, when intracavitary radium was first used. The Stockholm method was introduced in 1914, the Paris method in 1919, and the Manchester method in 1938. Because intracavitary radium does not provide an adequate cancericidal dose to the lymph nodes in the pelvis or to the lateral part of the parametria, the method of external radiotherapy was developed during the late 1920s and early 1930s, which led to improved results. Surgical treatment of carcinoma of the cervix has shown that even in stage I, about 15 to 25% of the lymph nodes show metastases. This is, of course, the background history of the routine treatment of the pelvic lymph nodes by radiotherapy, by surgery, or by a combination of the two. In later years, interest was focused on the treatment of the periaortic lymph nodes. There are conflicting opinions about the frequency of metastases to these nodes, both in early and later stages of the disease. In stage IIb, figures between 5 and 11% have been reported (1,2,5,12,13,15), although they are probably too low. In stage III, the figures vary between 35 and 50%.

Our treatment results in the period between the founding of Norwegian Radium Hospital and 1975 are shown in Fig. 1. In both stage I and Stage IIa, we prefer combined radium and surgical treatment, since our experience indicates that combined treatment gives better results. However, our results in the treatment of patients with stage III disease have been consistent over the years, even after the introduction of high-voltage machines in 1958.

Since 1970, we have performed extensive studies on the value of lymphography in predicting metastases. Our experiences with this technique in the treatment of stage Ib carcinoma of the cervix have been described in a series of articles (7–11). Kolbenstvedt (8) found that in a series of 300 patients on whom lymphography was performed both preoperatively and peroperatively, 36 of 77 cases with metastases were not detected by the lymphograms. These studies also convinced us that a complete dissection of all the lymph nodes in the pelvis is difficult, even with the use of peroperative lymphograms (10,11). We have not carried out studies of patients

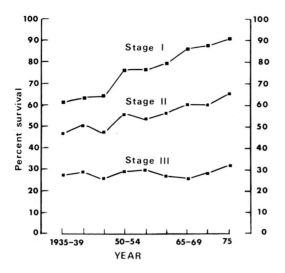

FIG. 1. Survival curves for women treated in Norwegian Radium Hospital for cervical cancer between 1935 and 1975.

with stage IIb or III disease, since we believe that no surgeon can perform a complete lymphadenectomy in the periaortic region and that lymphography cannot determine which patients would require some form of periaortic therapy in the lumbar region. Instead, we have found it expedient, because of the high percentage of lymph-node involvement in stages IIb and III reported in the literature, to irradiate the periaortic area.

In this chapter, we will present our preliminary findings and discuss the complications that occurred in 151 patients treated in this way during the period from 1975 to 1977.

MATERIAL AND METHODS

Table 1 provides details on the cases in the study. Most of the patients had stage IIb or III lesions, with only 13 having stage IV lesions. A total of 163 patients were originally included in the study, but 12 patients had to be withdrawn because of inability to tolerate the extended irradiation fields. Moreover, all 12 had complicating diseases and were older than the rest of the patients in the study. Thus,

TABLE 1. *163 cases treated in 1975 to 1977*

Stage	No. cases	No. withdrawn	No. evaluable
IIb	73	2	71
III	77	8	69
IV	13	2	11
Total	163	12	151

Observation time: 3 to 5 years.

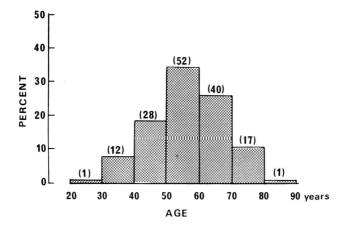

FIG. 2. Age distribution in series receiving periaortic irradiation.

151 patients were finally available for evaluation, all of whom were observed for 3 to 5 years.

Age Distribution

As can be seen from Fig. 2 and Table 2, a large percentage of the patients were from the older age group; such patients seem to consult their physicians later than younger women. The percentage of patients over 60 years of age increases with increasing disease stage. We also found that 75% of those withdrawn from the study were more than 60 years of age.

Histopathology

Distribution by histology is shown in Table 3. Approximately 90% of the patients had tumors of the squamous-cell group, while 5% had pure adenocarcinoma; there were 2 patients with adenosquamous carcinoma and 4 unclassified cases. We did not differentiate between small-cell carcinoma and large-cell carcinoma with or

TABLE 2. *Number and percentage of patients ≥ 60 yr*

Stage	Total no. patients	Patients ≥60 yr No.	%
IIb	71	22	31
III	69	30	43
IV	11	6	55
Withdrawn	12	9	75

TABLE 3. *Histopathology*

Type cancer	No.	%
Squamous cell carcinoma		
Highly to moderately differentiated	109	72.2
Poorly differentiated	28	18.5
Adenocarcinoma	8	5.3
Adenosquamous carcinoma	2	1.3
Unclassified	4	2.7
Total	151	100.0

without cornification, since in our experience such a subclassification has little bearing on the survival rate (3).

Treatment Schedule

In the years before the study, all patients received 5,000 rads to the pelvic wall through a field that extended to the bifurcation of the aorta and thus included the common iliac glands. In our series, we used a so-called "chimney field" (Fig. 3), which encompasses all the pelvic glands and the periaortic glands up to Th. XII.

The general treatment schedule at our hospital is as follows. Before actual treatment is begun, a work-up is performed, which includes a gynecologic examination under anesthesia. The size of the tumor is recorded. In stage IIb lesions we always record the size if the tumor extends out more than half way to the pelvic wall and if it is bilateral; bilaterality also is recorded in stage III lesions. Other standard examinations are also performed, including cystoscopy, chest X-ray, urography, venography, lymphangiography, whole blood count, and renal and liver function tests.

The details of the radiological treatment are shown in Table 4. External irradiation, 3,000 rads, is introduced through the anterior and posterior portals. The patient

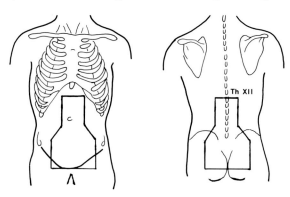

FIG. 3. "Chimney field" reaching Th. XII. When patient receives radium after 3,000 rads, central part of pelvis will be shielded.

TABLE 4. *Treatment for stage IIb, III, and IV carcinoma of the cervix*

Daily dose, 5 times a week	167 rads
Weekly dose	835 rads
Total dose	5,000 rads

Radium insertions after 3,000 rads; central shielding of the last 2,000 rads external irradiation. Radium dose = point A: 6,000–7,000 rads; point B: 800–1,500 rads.

is then examined to determine if it is possible to apply radium. The daily dose is 167 rads, five times a week, which equals a weekly dose of 835 rads. The total calculated dose to the pelvic wall and the periaortic region is 5,000 rads.

If it is feasible to apply radium after 3,000 rads, a modified Paris method is used, which gives a dose of about 6,000 to 7,000 rads to point A and about 800 to 1,500 rads to point B.

During the study, it was clear that we could not follow the above treatment schedule in all cases, especially in patients with stage III or IV disease, since an adequate insertion of radium in the vagina or cervix was not possible. In patients with stage IIb disease, as many as 97% were treated according to the given treatment schedule, while the figures for patients with stage III and stage IV disease were 67 and 55%, respectively. In some patients with very large stage III and stage IV tumors, the dose to the pelvis was increased to 6,000 rads (Table 5).

RESULTS

The 3- to 5-year survival rate in all 151 patients irrespective of the stage is shown in Table 6. It is evident that only patients whose treatment followed the treatment schedule achieved a reasonable 3- to 5-year survival rate of 54%. When external radiation could not be combined with intracavitary radium, only 4 of 22 patients survived during the period of observation. None of the patients with tumors necessitating a pelvic dose of 6,000 rads survived.

TABLE 5. *Treatment given in 151 cases available for evaluation*

	Stage					
	IIb		III		IV	
Treatment	No.	%	No.	%	No.	%
After schedule	69	97	46	67	6	55
External radiation only, 5,000 rads	2	3	19	27	1	9
External radiation, pelvic dose 6,000 rads	0	0	4	6	4	36

If we break up the group in the series according to the different stages, then in Table 7 we see the results of the 71 patients with stage IIb tumors. The crude survival rate was 58%. Once more it is evident that if radium cannot be applied, the prognosis is poor.

We also studied the value of differentiating between patients that had an extension only to the medial half and those having an extension to the lateral half of one or both parametria. At the same time, we sought to determine whether patients with a unilateral tumor had a better prognosis than patients with a bilateral tumor (Table 8). The results are quite clear: The larger the tumor, the poorer the prognosis. In Stage III, patients with unilateral tumors fare better than those with bilateral tumors.

In the 69 patients with stage III lesions, the crude survival rate during the observation period was 36% (Table 9); two patients died from intercurrent disease. Once again it was observed that patients having tumors that made it possible to combine radium with external irradiation had a better prognosis than those receiving external irradiation alone. Increasing the pelvic dose to 6,000 rads seemed to have little effect.

TABLE 6. *Treatment schedule and survival rate*

Treatment	Total no.	Survival rate	
		No.	%
3,000 rads "chimney field"; radium, 2,000 rads shielded	121	65	54
External radiation only, 5,000 rads	22	4	18
Periaortic dose 5,000 rads; pelvic dose 6,000 rads	8	0	0
Total	151	69	46

TABLE 7. *Treatment and survival rate in 71 stage IIb cases*

Treatment	Total no.	Survival rate	
		No.	%
After schedule	69	41[a]	59
External radiation only, 5,000 rads	2	0	0
Periaortic dose 5,000 rads; pelvic dose 6,000 rads	0	0	0
Total	71	41	58

[a]One patient died from intercurrent disease.
Observation time: 3 to 5 years.

TABLE 8. *Parametrial extension and prognosis in 71 stage IIb cases and 64 stage III cases*

Extension	Total no.	Survival rate	
		No.	%
Stage IIb			
Medial half	22	15	68
Lateral half	49	28	57
Stage III			
One side	24	11	46
Both sides	40	11	28

TABLE 9. *Treatment and survival in 69 stage III cases*

Treatment	Total no.	Survival rate	
		No.	%
After schedule	46	21[a]	46
External radiation only, 5,000 rads	19	4[b]	21
Periaortic dose 5,000 rads; pelvic dose 6,000 rads	4	0	0
Total	69	25	36

[a]One patient died from intercurrent disease.
[b]One patient died from intercurrent disease.
Observation time: 3 to 5 years.

Only 11 patients with stage IV disease were evaluable. To this date, 3 of the 11 remain alive; all received both radium and external radiation (Table 10).

Complications

The observed complications are listed in Table 11. The most common complication was persistent diarrhea, which occurred in 18% of the cases. By persistent we mean that during the follow-up the patient complained of diarrhea more than 2 months after treatment. Sometimes the diarrhea lasted up to 6 months. Other complications, which are not considered serious, are nausea, vomiting, and/or diarrhea during therapy. In some cases, intravenous fluids had to be administered to compensate for electrolyte and water loss. In 2 patients, we observed intestinal obstruction and perforation, and 1 patient died. Surprisingly, the most common major complication was gastric ulcer. Two of the 7 patients listed in Table 11 had had gastric ulcer for some years before treatment. Of the 7 patients, 6 are now dead. However, it should be emphasized that only 2 died from complications; the other

TABLE 10. *Treatment and survival in 11 stage IV cases*

Treatment	Total no.	No. alive
After schedule	6	3
External radiation only, 5,000 rads	1	0
Periaortic dose 5,000 rads; pelvic dose 6,000 rads	4	0

TABLE 11. *Most likely complications from irradiation*

Complication	No.	%	Dead
Gastric ulcer	7	4.6	6[a]
Intestinal obstruction and perforation	2	1.3	1
Persistent diarrhea	27	17.9	0
Other, not serious	20	13.2	0

[a]Only two died from complications. See text.

4 died from a recurrence of the cancer. The gastric ulcer was detected either by X-ray examination of the stomach a few months after treatment was finished (3 cases) or by autopsy (1 case). The last patient had a tumor that never showed primary healing, as well as liver metastases.

DISCUSSION

There are several approaches to the problem of the treatment of periaortic lymph nodes. After the invention of lymphography, several studies seemed to indicate that this method of visualizing metastases is reliable (4,6,8). However, other studies, e.g., those of Brown et al. (5) or Ballon et al. (2), clearly demonstrated that this is not so. There is a relatively high number of both false-negative and false-positive lymphograms, which is in complete agreement with our studies on the accuracy of pelvic lymphography in the treatment of stage Ib cervical cancer. Between 1970 and 1973, 300 consecutive patients received combined surgery and radiotherapy, including pelvic lymphadenectomy under peroperative lymphographic control. A total of 9,187 lymph nodes were removed, of which 770 were found with the aid of peroperative radiograms. Of the 300 patients, 77 proved to have pelvic lymph-node metastases, whereas 36 had false-negative lymphograms. Of the remaining 223, 15 had false-positive lymphograms. Therefore, we believe that one cannot rely on lymphography to determine which patients should have periaortic irradiation.

The best way of detecting periaortic lymph-node metastases is to perform both lymphography and periaortic lymph-node dissection. However, it is extremely difficult to remove all the lymph nodes around the aorta, considerably more difficult than to perform a complete dissection in the pelvic region. Piver and Barlow (13) reported on this combined procedure in 1973. Patients who had positive nodes and received postoperative external irradiation showed considerable intestinal complications. Wharton et al. (15) observed similar results in a series at their hospital. However, Tewfik et al. (14) concluded that it can be expected that periaortic irradiation can control some metastases with a rather acceptable risk. The same conclusion was reached by Ballon et al. (2), whose series was relatively large because it included some large Ib and IIa lesions. However, Ballon et al. do not provide the exact percentage of involved periaortic nodes but include the common iliac nodes in the periaortic group. If one must arrive at any conclusion about the combination of periaortic lymphadenectomy and external irradiation, it seems from the literature that the number of complications can be reduced by more conservative radiotherapy. The higher the dose to the periaortic region, the more complications arise. Ballon et al. used a retroperitoneal approach in lymphadenectomy, believing that this will help reduce the number of complications.

Our own approach has been conservative. We do not believe that periaortic sampling of nodes will determine the exact percentage of nodes involved. Furthermore, we believe that considerable experience is needed to carry out a complete dissection in this area. Nevertheless, there is little doubt that with increasing disease stage there is a higher percentage of node involvement in the periaortic region. We therefore find it expedient to include this region in the external radiotherapy field. We can only report 3- to 5-year survival rates. Using an actuarial method of calculating the survival curve and comparing data from the series 1971 to 1973 with the series from 1975 to 1977, we find no increase in survival in the latter series. However, before reaching a final conclusion, we will continue our series for several more years to gather more data. We suggest a maximum dose of 4,000 to 4,500 rads to the periaortic region rather than the 6,000 rads that has been recommended. We also do not recommend increasing the pelvic dose to 6,000 rads, since none of the patients who received this dose in our series has survived. It must also be concluded that only in those cases in which it is possible to treat the primary tumor by intracavitary sources can the results be expected to improve by including the periaortic region in the radiation field. External irradiation by itself cannot compete with combined intracavitary and external irradiation.

REFERENCES

1. Averette, H. E., Dudan, R. C., and Ford, J. H., Jr. (1972): Exploratory celiotomy for surgical staging of cervical cancer. *Am. J. Obstet. Gynecol.*, 113:1090–1094.
2. Ballon, S. C., Berman, M. L., Lagasse, L. D., Petrilli, E. S., and Castaldo, T. W. (1981): Survival after extraperitoneal pelvic and paraaortic lymphadenectomy and radiation therapy in cervical carcinoma. *Obstet. Gynecol.*, 57(1):90–95.
3. Beecham, J. B., Halvorsen, T., Kolbenstvedt, A. (1978): Histologic classification, lymph node metastases, and patient survival in stage IB cervical carcinoma: An analysis of 245 uniformly treated cases. *Gynecol. Oncol.*, 6:95–105.
4. Brady, L. W. (1975): Advances in the management of gynecologic cancer. Radiation therapy. *Cancer*, 36:661–665.
5. Brown, R. C., Buchsbaum, H. J., Tewfik, H. H., and Platz, C. E. (1979): Accuracy of lymphangiography in the diagnosis of paraaortic lymph node metastases from carcinoma of the cervix. *Obstet. Gynecol.*, 54(5):571–575.
6. Emami, B., Watring, W. G., Tak, W., Anderson, B., and Piro, A. J. (1980): Para-aortic lymph node radiation in advanced cervical cancer. *Int. J. Radiat., Oncol. Biol. Phys.*, 6(9):1237–1241.

7. Kolbenstvedt, A. (1974): A critical evaluation of foot lymphography in the demonstration of the regional lymph nodes of the uterine cervix. *Gynecol. Oncol.*, 2:34–38.

8. Kolbenstvedt, A. (1975): Lymphography in the diagnosis of metastases from carcinoma of the cervix stages I and II. *Acta Radiol.* [Diagn.] (Stock.), 16:81–97.

9. Kolbenstvedt, A., and Knudsen, O. S. (1974): A method for lymphographic and histologic correlation. Experience from 300 patients treated by pelvic lymphadenectomy. *Gynecol. Oncol.*, 2:9–23.

10. Kolbenstvedt, A., and Kolstad, P. (1974): Pelvic lymph node dissection under peroperative lymphographic control. *Gynecol. Oncol.*, 2:39–59.

11. Kolbenstvedt, A., and Kolstad, P. (1976): The difficulties of complete pelvic lymph node dissection in radical hysterectomy for carcinoma of the cervix. *Gynec. Oncol.*, 4:244–254.

12. Nelson, J. H., Jr., Macasaet, M. A., Lu, T., Bohorquez, J. F., Smart, G. E., Nicastri, A. D., and Walton, L. A. (1974): Incidence and significance of para-aortic lymph node metastases in late invasive carcinoma of the cervix. *Am. J. Obstet. Gynecol.*, 118:749–755.

13. Piver, M. S., and Barlow, J. J. (1974): Para-aortic lymphadenectomy in staging patients with advanced local cervical cancer. *Obstet. Gynecol.*, 34:544–548.

14. Tewfik, H., Buchsbaum, H., Latourette, H., Lifshitz, S., and Tewfik, F. (1980): Paraaortic lymph node irradiated in carcinoma of the cervix after exploratory laparotomy and biopsy confirmed aortic nodes. *Proc. Am. Assoc. Cancer Res.*, 21:398.

15. Wharton, J. T., Jones, H. W., III, Day, T. G., Jr., Rutledge, F. N., and Fletcher, G. H. (1977): Preirradiation celiotomy and extended field irradiation for invasive carcinoma of the cervix. *Obstet. Gynecol.*, 49:333–338.

Recent Clinical Developments in Gynecologic Oncology, edited by C. Paul Morrow, et al.
Raven Press, New York © 1983.

Prevention of Venous Thromboembolism After Pelvic Surgery

John Bonnar

Department of Obstetrics and Gynaecology, University of Dublin, Trinity College Unit, Rotunda Hospital, Dublin 1, Ireland

Postoperative thrombosis with embolism is one of the most common causes of death following pelvic surgery. Since the majority of patients with fatal pulmonary embolism die within 1 hour, without diagnosis and treatment the number of deaths will not be greatly reduced by improvements in treatment. In the United States, the total incidence of pulmonary embolism is estimated to be 600,000 cases per year (7,16). Pulmonary embolism is the sole cause of death in approximately 100,000 patients and a major contributory cause in another 100,000, making pulmonary embolism the third most frequent cause of death in the United States (16).

A decrease in the number of deaths from venous thromboembolism can be achieved by taking into account the predisposing factors and by the selective use of effective prophylactic measures. The patient undergoing surgery for gynaecological malignancy is in an especially high-risk category for postoperative thrombosis and embolism. Pulmonary embolism, albeit the most serious complication of venous thromboembolism, is only part of the clinical problem. Chronic venous insufficiency leading to oedema, pain, eczema, and ulceration of the legs is a common sequela to leg-vein thrombosis (11,12).

The advent of new objective techniques for diagnosing venous thrombosis has provided a wealth of information on its natural history following surgery and a reliable means of evaluating methods of prophylaxis and treatment. When pulmonary embolism occurs, the source of the thrombi is generally the deep veins of the legs and pelvis, i.e., the popliteal, femoral or iliac veins (Figs. 1 and 2). The lungs are natural filters for small venous clots, which are readily lysed by the active fibrinolytic system in the pulmonary vascular endothelium. Large thrombi or a shower of small clots can, however, overwhelm the ability of the lung to fragment and dissolve them.

INCIDENCE OF THROMBOSIS AFTER GYNAECOLOGICAL SURGERY

The incidence of thrombosis after gynaecological surgery has been evaluated by the I^{125} fibrinogen uptake test, which is highly sensitive for detecting and localizing

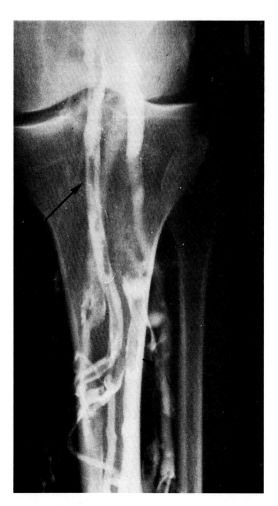

FIG. 1. Phlebography showing deep veins of calf with thrombi extending into popliteal vein below knee.

deep-vein thrombosis in the lower limbs (2,15). I^{125} fibrinogen studies, along with phlebography, have shown that the process of thrombosis usually originates in the calf veins and generally starts either during or immediately after surgery (15). In approximately 20% of patients who develop thrombosis in the calf veins, thrombi extend into the popliteal, femoral, and iliac veins (Fig. 3). In this group with extending thrombosis, pulmonary embolism occurs in almost 50% of cases but will prove fatal in only a small number. Where the thrombi remain confined to the calf, they are of little clinical significance, and for all practical purposes emboli do not occur (Fig. 4). Using the radioactive fibrinogen method, the overall incidence of subclinical leg-vein thrombosis following gynaecological procedures has been shown to be between 5 and 35% (2,15). As shown in Fig. 5, the incidence is highest in patients undergoing surgical treatment for malignant disease, particularly carcinoma of the vulva and ovary.

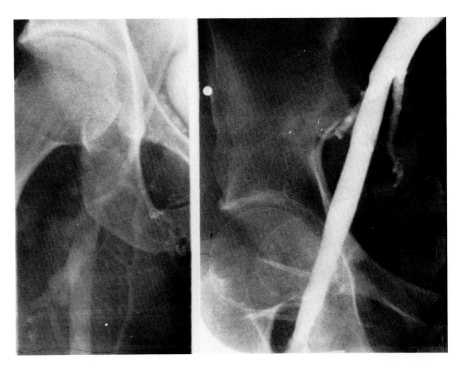

FIG. 2. Venous thrombosis obstructing ileofemoral segment **(right)** and normal phlebogram **(left)**.

PREVENTION OF VENOUS THROMBOEMBOLISM

General

The programme for the prevention of venous thrombosis should begin when the patient is first seen in the out-patient department. Certain patients are particularly at risk from this complication (see Table 1). High-risk factors are malignant disease, advanced years, a previous history of thromboembolism, obesity, varicose veins, and oestrogen therapy. The incidence of deep-vein thrombosis is increased fourfold in women undergoing surgery who have been taking combined oestrogen-progestogen oral contraceptives (14); if the contraceptives are discontinued 6 to 8 weeks before surgery, this additional hazard is greatly reduced.

Hospitalisation for longer than 1 or 2 days before surgery increases the hazard of thrombosis. All necessary preoperative investigations and consultations should therefore be completed if possible as out-patient procedures prior to admission, and the patient should be admitted the day before surgery whenever possible. In cases where a patient suffers from chronic respiratory disease, preoperative physiotherapy before admission and cessation of smoking are recommended. Full movement of

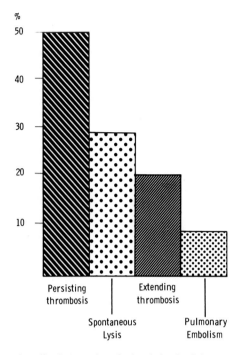

FIG. 3. Behaviour of thrombi in leg veins after pelvic surgery, diagnosed and monitored by I^{125} fibrinogen technique. In approximately 20% of patients who develop thrombi in calf veins, thrombotic process extends into popliteal, femoral, or iliac veins. In 50% of patients with extending thrombosis, pulmonary emboli can be detected.

the diaphragm is of physiological importance in maintaining good venous return from the lower limbs and pelvis.

During surgery, certain precautions are advisable to reduce venous pooling in the pelvic veins and lower limbs. The 20° to 30° tilt of the patient, which is common during gynaecological operations, improves venous blood flow from the legs. The patient's heels should be supported during abdominal surgery to protect the soleal veins in the calf from the pressure of the operating table. Pressure on the inferior vena cava caused by excessive abdominal packing should be avoided, particularly during prolonged surgical procedures. Care must also be taken to avoid unnecessary pressure or trauma to large blood vessels with retractors. Strict asepsis, the gentle handling of tissue, and good haemostasis are all of vital importance, since they will affect the recovery and mobility of the patient in the postoperative period.

After the operation, active leg exercises after recovery from anaesthesia are recommended, as well as early ambulation, beginning on the day after surgery. In the postoperative period, early ambulation often means that the patient is transferred from the bed to a chair with knees and thighs flexed—more aptly termed "early angulation"—a position that seriously impedes venous return from the legs. In high-risk patients, elevation of the foot of the bed by at least 15° improves venous flow from the lower limbs and is helpful especially in patients who have had radical vulvectomy.

Specific Measurements for Preventing Venous Thrombosis

For patients undergoing surgical treatment for gynaecological malignant disease, prophylaxis is essential. Table 1 shows the incidence of thromboembolic complications in low-risk gynaecological patients compared with high-risk patients.

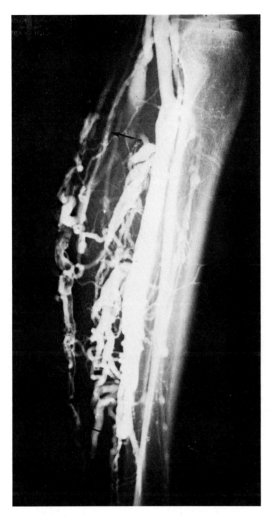

FIG. 4. Venous plexus of calf showing small, clinically insignificant thrombus in one of soleal veins. Venous plexus should be protected from effects of pressure from operating table during surgery.

A number of methods are available for preventing venous thrombosis and pulmonary embolism. They include low-dosage administration of heparin, dextran, and oral anticoagulants, pneumatic compression of the calf, and electrical stimulation of the calf muscles.

LOW-DOSE HEPARIN

Heparin is used prophylactically in a dose of 5,000 units administered subcutaneously 2 hr prior to surgery and then repeated at either 8- or 12-hr intervals after surgery. Both regimens effectively reduce the frequency of postoperative venous thromboembolism (9,12). Our own studies (4) have shown that the bioavailability of heparin is greater from the sodium salt of heparin than from the calcium salt. If calcium heparin is used, an 8-hr regimen is advisable, whereas a 12-hr regimen is adequate with sodium heparin (Fig. 6).

TABLE 1. *Assessment of risk of venous thromboembolism in gynaecological patients*

	Low risk[a] (%)	Moderate risk[b] (%)	High risk[c] (%)
Calf-vein thrombosis	<3	1–30	30–60
Proximal-vein thrombosis	<1	2–8	6–12
Pulmonary embolism	<0.01	0.1–0.7	1–2

[a]Under 40 years; operative procedures less than 30 min; no immobilization.
[b]Over 40 years; oestrogen therapy; operative procedures longer than 30 min; varicose veins; obesity; postoperative infection.
[c]Previous thromboembolism; abdominal or pelvic surgery for malignant disease; immobilization.

Prophylaxis with heparin should be continued during the entire high-risk period, which usually lasts 7 days or until the patient is fully ambulatory. Treatment with low-dose heparin decreases the frequency of small thrombi in the calf veins and the frequency of proximal-vein thrombi and major pulmonary emboli (10,11). Treatment with low-dose heparin, expecially on an 8-hr regimen, is associated with an increase in the incidence of wound haematomas (9).

Use of Subcutaneous Heparin

Particular care is required in the instruction of both the nursing staff and patients in the use of subcutaneous heparin. A concentrated aqueous solution of 25,000 units of heparin in 1 ml should be used, and a tuberculin-type syringe and a 25- or 26-gauge needle 1.5 cm in length. A fold of skin is gently raised in the flank on the lateral aspect of the anterior abdominal wall and the needle inserted full

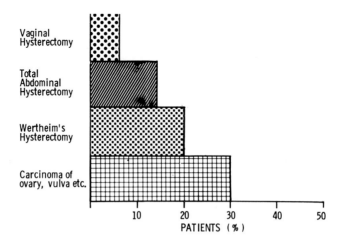

FIG. 5. Incidence of deep venous thrombosis following pelvic surgery as shown by radioactive I[125] fibrinogen studies and phlebography. [From Walsh et al. (15), with permission.]

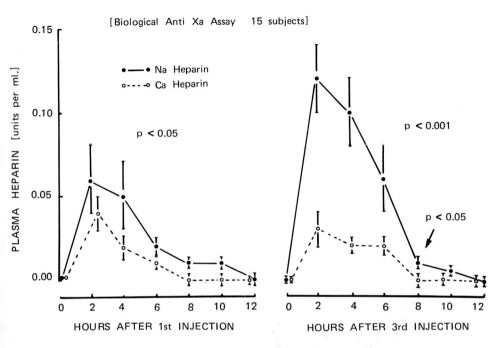

FIG. 6. Comparison of plasma heparin levels after subcutaneous sodium and calcium heparin, 5,000 units every 12 hr.

depth directly at a right angle to the skin. The needle is slowly removed at the same angle as inserted, taking care to avoid damaging the skin and subcutaneous fat at the injection site. The injection site should not be rubbed or massaged. Subcutaneous heparin should not be given in the arms or legs; apart from being more painful and causing bruising, the limb movements may accelerate the rate of absorption of the heparin.

PROPHYLAXIS WITH DEXTRAN

We have shown that 1 litre of dextran 70 administered during and immediately after surgery over a 6-hr period that started after the induction of anaesthesia produced a highly significant reduction in the frequency of postoperative thrombosis after pelvic surgery (3,5). In our study, we found that the frequency of thrombosis after abdominal hysterectomy in benign conditions was more than twice that occurring after vaginal hysterectomy for similar pathology. A similar finding was also reported by Bernstein et al (2). Likewise, in patients undergoing Wertheim's operation, perioperative infusion of 1 litre of dextran 70 reduced the incidence of leg-vein thrombosis detected in I^{125} fibrinogen from 33 to 5% (3,6). When given as described, dextran 70 is present in the circulation for more than 7 days, and its antithrombotic action appears to be through the effects of dextran on blood flow, platelets, coagulation factors V and VIII, and fibrinolysis (3) (Fig. 7). If dextran

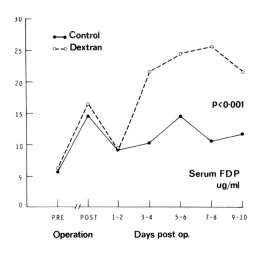

FIG. 7. Effect of dextran 70 on fibrinolytic system during and after radical pelvic surgery (Wertheim's hysterectomy) as shown by higher levels of serum fibrin degradation products (FDP); mean results in 16 patients in control group and 16 patients given 1 litre of dextran 70 during and after surgery. Presence of dextran in circulation may accelerate presence of spontaneous lysis of any thrombi.

of lower molecular weight is used, such as dextran 40, the dextran will be excreted more quickly, and an infusion of 500 ml should be repeated daily for 2 to 5 days.

Dextran 70 has been reported to be as effective as low-dose heparin for preventing fatal pulmonary embolism after general surgical procedures (8,13). It should be noted that dextran and heparin should not be given together, since the combination has a synergistic effect on blood clotting and consequently the risk of bleeding is greatly increased.

ORAL ANTICOAGULANTS

To be effective at the time of surgery, oral anticoagulant therapy should be instituted at least 24 to 48 hr before surgery. When a patient is under the influence of oral anticoagulants at the time of the operation, the risk of bleeding at and immediately after surgery is increased. To avoid the hazard of bleeding, oral anticoagulants have been started 2 to 3 days after surgery in doses that prolong the prothrombin time to 1.5 to 2 times the control levels.

This approach on its own will not prevent the formation of venous thrombi, which occur at or immediately after surgery. It may, however, effectively inhibit the spread of the thrombotic process and thereby reduce the frequency of clinically significant venous thromboemboli. In the author's opinion, the incidence of bleeding complications with oral anticoagulants is too high to justify the routine use of this method of prophylaxis in gynaecological surgery.

PHYSICAL METHODS OF PROPHYLAXIS

The use of pneumatic compression of the leg and electrical stimulation of the calf muscles has been evaluated to a limited extent with respect to the prevention of venous thrombosis. Further investigation is necessary before their use can be recommended to replace either low-dose heparin or dextran prophylaxis. In cases where dextran and heparin are contraindicated, the physical methods of prophylaxis should be considered. In high-risk patients, physical methods can be used in combination with dextran or low-dose heparin.

CHOICE OF METHOD OF PROPHYLAXIS

Patients suffering from gynaecological malignancy who are undergoing surgical treatment must be considered at high risk to thromboembolic complications. If such patients are unprotected, they have a 30 to 60% chance of developing venous thrombosis in the legs, a 6 to 12% chance of developing proximal-vein thrombosis, and a 1 to 2% chance of developing fatal pulmonary embolism (9). Based on our experience over the last 10 years, the following regimens are used:

1. Dextran 70: perioperative infusion of 1 litre starting after induction of anaesthesia.
2. Heparin: 5,000 units of sodium heparin at 12-hr intervals by subcutaneous injection.

Regimen 1 is used in patients under 60 years of age who have no evidence of any cardiac or renal abnormality and no history of allergy and whose operative procedure will not exceed 2 hr. Dextran 70 is not used when it is likely that the patient's postoperative immobilization is likely to exceed more than 5 days.

Regimen 2 is used in all patients over the age of 60 undergoing major gynaecological surgery, patients under 60 with any evidence of cardiac or renal impairment, patients with a history of allergy, patients undergoing operative procedures longer than 2 hr, and patients who are likely to be immobilised for more than 5 days after the surgical procedure, e.g., radical vulvectomy.

FIBRINOLYTIC DRUGS AND VENOUS THROMBOEMBOLISM

Despite the use of effective methods for preventing deep-vein thrombosis, it will still occur in a small percentage of patients. No method of prophylaxis will provide 100% protection against venous thromboembolism. The use of streptokinase or urokinase to treat postoperative leg-vein thrombosis is limited by the substantial risk of haemorrhage where such treatment is used in the first 10 days after surgery. Fibrin plays an essential role in wound healing, and all the fibrin in the body will be broken down by streptokinase or urokinase. When a deep-vein thrombosis occurs in the thigh or pelvic veins as a late complication, e.g., after 14 days, treatment with streptokinase can be considered. If haemorrhage from the operation site develops, treatment must be discontinued. A recent report from Sweden (1) suggests that fibrinolytic treatment is by no means certain to prevent the development of the postthrombotic syndrome. At an average of 29 months after streptokinase treatment for a proven deep-vein thrombosis, only 2 of 35 patients were without symptoms and signs of venous insufficiency (1).

CONCLUSION

Deep-vein thrombosis and pulmonary embolism are potential complications in all patients undergoing surgery for gynaecological malignancy. Clinical diagnosis of thrombosis, which is often unreliable, has now been superseded by objective techniques that enable the precise location and extent of the thrombotic process to be more accurately determined. The availability of these methods to gynaecologists allows early diagnosis and the institution of treatment to prevent the extension of the thrombotic process and embolism.

However, the most important approach to this serious complication is prophylaxis. The administration of dextran 70 during the critical period of surgery and immediately after or the use of low-dose heparin are recommended in all patients undergoing major surgery for gynaecological malignancy.

REFERENCES

1. Albrechtson, U., Anderson, J., Einarsson, E., Eklof, B., and Norgren, L. (1981): Streptokinase treatment of deep vein thrombosis and the post-thrombotic syndrome. *Arch. Surg.*, 116:33–37.
2. Bernstein, K., Ulmsten, U., Astedt, B., Jacobsson, L., and Mattson, S. (1980): Incidence of thrombosis after gynaecological surgery evaluated by an improved I[125] fibrinogen uptake test. *Angiology*, 31:606–613.
3. Bonnar, J. (1977): The use of Dextran for the prophylaxis of post-operative thromboembolic complications. In: *The Detection and Treatment of Thromboembolism*, edited by C. D. Forbes and N. Mackay, pp. 129–136. Trust for Education and Research in Therapeutics, London.
4. Bonnar, J. (1981): Haemostasis and coagulation disorders in pregnancy. In: *Haemostasis and Thrombosis*, edited by A. L. Bloom and D. P. Thomas, pp. 454–471. Churchill Livingstone, London and New York.
5. Bonnar, J., and Walsh, J. (1972): Prevention of thrombosis after pelvic surgery by British Dextran 70. *Lancet*, 1:614–616.
6. Bonnar, J., Walsh, J. J., Haddon, M., Fairweather, J., and Denson, K. W. E. (1973): Coagulation system changes induced by pelvic surgery and the effect of Dextran 70. 7th Conference of the European Society for the Microcirculation. *Bibl. Anat.*, 12:351–355.
7. Coon, W. W. (1977): Epidemiology of venous thromboembolism. *Ann. Surg.*, 186(2):149–164.
8. Gruber, U. F., Saldeen, T., Brokopt, T., and Eklof, B. (1980): Incidences of fatal post-operative pulmonary embolism after prophylaxis with Dextran 70 and low-dose Heparin: An international multi-centre study. *Br. Med. J.*, 280:69–72.
9. Hirsh, J. (1981): Choosing the best of old and new ways to prevent venous thrombosis. *J. Cardio. Med.*, July:691–701.
10. Hirsh, J., et al. (1975): Low-dose Heparin prophylaxis for venous thromboembolism. In: *Prophylactic Therapy for Deep Venous Thrombosis and Pulmonary Embolism*, edited by J. Fratantoni. D. H. E. W. Publication No. (N.I.H.) 76–866, p. 254.
11. Kakkar, V. V. (1975): Efficacy of low-dose Heparin in preventing post-operative fatal pulmonary embolism: Results of an international multi-centre trial. In: *Prophylactic Therapy for Deep Venous Thrombosis and Pulmonary Embolism*, edited by J. Fratantoni. D. H. E. W. Publication No. (N.I.H.) 76-866, p. 207.
12. Kakkar, V. V. (1981): Prevention of venous thromboembolism. In: *Haemostasis and Thrombosis*, edited by A. L. Bloom and D. P. Thomas, pp. 669–683. Churchill Livingstone, London and New York.
13. Kline, A., Hughes, L. E., Campbell, H., William, A., et al. (1975): Dextran 70 in prophylaxis of thromboembolic disease after surgery—a clinically oriented randomised double-blind trial. *Br. Med. J.*, 2:109–112.
14. Vessey, M. P. (1973): The epidemiology of venous thromboembolism. In: *Recent Advances in Thrombosis*, edited by L. Poller, pp. 39–58. Churchill Livingstone, London and New York.
15. Walsh, J. J., Bonnar, J., and Wright, F. W. (1974): A study of pulmonary embolism and deep-vein thrombosis after major gynaecological surgery using labelled fibrinogen, phlebography and lung scanning. *J. Obstet. Gynaecol. Br. Commonw.*, 81:311–319.
16. Wilson, J. E. (1981): Pulmonary embolism: diagnosis and treatment. *Clin. Notes Respir. Dis.*, 20:3–13.

Recent Clinical Developments in Gynecologic Oncology, edited by C. Paul Morrow, et al. Raven Press, New York © 1983.

Recent Advances in Trophoblastic Disease

C. Paul Morrow and John B. Schlaerth

Department of Obstetrics and Gynecology, University of Southern California School of Medicine, Los Angeles, California 90033

During the past few years, much knowledge has been contributed to the subject of trophoblastic tumors, leading to improvements in both diagnosis and prognosis. The specific areas of progress that will be discussed in this chapter are (a) the etiology and classification of hydatid mole, (b) the problems of managing hydatid mole, (c) the postmolar serum human chorionic gonadotropin (hCG) regression curve, (d) hormonal contraception, (e) repeat curettage, (f) prophylactic chemotherapy, (g) indications for the treatment of postmolar trophoblastic disease (PMTD), (h) treatment regimens for nonmetastatic postmolar trophoblastic disease, and (i) new treatment regimens for metastatic trophoblastic disease.

ETIOLOGY AND CLASSIFICATION OF HYDATID MOLE

Four categories of molar pregnancy, characterized by the degree of swelling of the placental villi, have been recognized (26): (a) the complete hydatidiform mole, (b) the partial mole accompanied by a fetus, (c) the transitional mole (a "blighted ovum" with swollen villi), and (d) the partial or complete hydatid mole concomitant with a separate pregnancy. Table 1 compares the features of these various forms according to the descriptions of Vassilakos et al. (26) and Szulman and Surti (22). Perhaps the most important consideration regarding these different types of molar pregnancy is the risk of trophoblastic malignancy, which has been reasonably well defined with respect to complete moles (Table 2). While the malignancy risk for partial moles is undoubtedly less, it appears to be higher than that for nonmolar pregnancy. In addition to a number of case reports (11,23), Goldstein, et al. (9) reported a series of 23 patients with partial moles none of whom required chemotherapy, and Szulman et al. (24) noted only 1 case of malignancy among 13 patients with partial moles.

It is tempting to speculate about the reasons why partial moles have a lower malignancy risk than complete moles. An obvious explanation may be the observed difference in the degree of trophoblastic hyperplasia, anaplasia, or immaturity. Another factor may be genetic. Partial moles are usually 69XX or 69XY, while complete moles are almost invariably 46XX, although 46XY karyotype has been

TABLE 1. *Comparison of various types of molar pregnancy*

	Complete	Incomplete	Transitional
Synonyms	True; classic	Partial	Blighted ovum
Villi	All swollen	Some normal	Some normal
Capillaries	Few; no fetal RBCs	Many; fetal RBCs	Present
Trophoblastic hyperplasia	Marked	Minimal to moderate	Normal or hypoplastic
Embryo	No cord, amnion or fetus	Abnormal fetus	Amnion; stunted embryo
Gestational age	8–16 weeks	10–22 weeks	First trimester
hCG titers	High	High to low	Low
Malignant potential	High	Low	Slight, if any
Karyotype	Predominantly 46XX	Triploid	Trisomic; triploid

RBC: red blood cells.

reported (16). Furthermore, the chromosomes of complete moles are entirely of paternal origin (12), apparently as a result of fertilization by 1 (23X) or 2 (23X; 23Y) haploid spermatozoa without participation of the ovum nucleus.

PROBLEMS IN DIAGNOSIS AND MANAGEMENT OF HYDATID MOLAR PREGNANCY

The woman with a molar pregnancy usually presents as a threatened abortion, with a uterus greater than 12 weeks gestational size (often large for menstrual dates), hyperemesis, or midtrimester toxemia. Pregnant women with any of these features should be evaluated by ultrasound regardless of whether or not fetal heart tones are present. The differential diagnoses are given in Table 3. Once the diagnosis is confirmed by ultrasound or amniography (Table 4), evacuation of the uterus is carried out by suction curettage (Table 5). In the postevacuation period, the patient must be observed for acute pulmonary insufficiency. In our experience, this occurs

TABLE 2. *Reported incidence of PMTD in United States*

Ref.	Total no. cases	NMTD (%)	MTD (%)	All TD (%)
9	858	14.7	4.0	18.6
7	337	16.6	3.5	20.2
4	51	19.6	2.0	21.6
14	121	23.1	3.3	26.4
13	127	26.0	3.1	29.1
10	212	26.4	5.7	32.0

NMTD: nonmetastatic trophoblastic disease, MTD: metastatic trophoblastic disease, TD: trophoblastic disease.

TABLE 3. *Differential diagnosis of molar pregnancy*

Early intrauterine gestation with
    Englarging myoma
    Ovarian neoplasm
    Polyhydramnios

Multifetal gestation

Fetus and mole

Intrauterine fetal death

Wrong menstrual dates

only in patients with a uterus greater than 16 weeks gestational size and is usually the result of fluid overload in the presence of a compromised cardiac reserve (6,25). The administration of oxygen and a diuretic is usually sufficient therapy. A second early postevacuation complication is infection, accompanied by positive blood cultures in 10% of cases.

Suction curettage is the single most effective means of evacuating molar pregnancy regardless of the uterine size. Hysterotomy is indicated only in the case of hydatid mole with a live fetus more than 24 weeks gestational age or severe preeclampsia. The use of vaginal prostaglandins or other oxytocics should be limited to the patient with a second-trimester fetus and mole. These agents take up to 24 hr to produce abortion and must usually be followed by curettage to complete evacuation of the molar tissue.

POSTMOLAR hCG REGRESSION CURVE

Analysis of weekly serum β-hCG levels after the onset of molar pregnancy has identified two distinct groups of patients: one characterized by a progressive decline in the serum hCG to normal (14), as shown in Fig. 1, and one characterized by an early deviation producing a significant plateau or rise in the serum hCG titer (19), as shown in Fig. 2. Patients in the latter group have either incompletely evacuated moles or trophoblastic neoplasia (invasive mole or choriocarcinoma). However, we have not found molar tissue at curettage in patients experiencing a plateau or rise in hCG titer under these circumstances and can only conclude that all have trophoblastic neoplasia. This is further supported by our experience that every patient

TABLE 4. *Amniography for diagnosis of hydatid mole*

Place spinal needle into uterus through abdominal wall

Aspirate
    Amniotic fluid indicates presence of fetus

    If no amniotic fluid obtained, inject radioopaque dye,
        about 1cc/week gestational size; take anterior-posterior
        radiograph

TABLE 5. *Method of suction curettage*

Done in operating room under general anesthesia
Blood available
Large i.v. line in place
Cervical dilation usually easy or unnecessary
Insert large (12-mm) vacuum curet with vacuum off
Fenestration should be just inside (above) internal os
Turn suction to 1 atm pressure
Start pitocin drip
Rotate curet to right and left
Follow with gentle mechanical curettage using large curet

---

undergoing hysterectomy for persistent abnormal titers, with or without chemo-therapy, has had invasive mole or choriocarcinoma identified histologically. This does not mean that treatment is necessarily warranted in all cases with an abnormal hCG regression curve, but it permits early and accurate recognition of the population at risk. We have elected to treat nearly all such patients on a routine basis, since patient compliance is poor even over the course of 6 months.

HORMONAL CONTRACEPTION

The avoidance of pregnancy during the period of postmolar follow-up, at least until titer remission occurs, has been universally recommended to avoid confusing

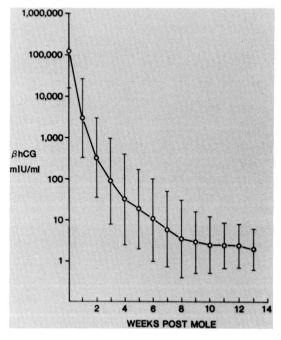

FIG. 1. Normal serum β-hCG regression curve following molar pregnancy. Curve depicts mean values and 95% confidence limits. (From Schlaerth et al., ref. 19, with permission.)

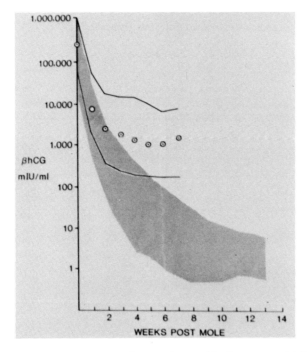

FIG. 2. Stippled area represents normal regression corridor for serum β-hCG. Mean values (○) and 95% confidence limits for serum hCG values from patients having abnormal regression curves are superimposed. Curves separate 5 to 6 weeks after evacuation. (From Schlaerth et al., ref. 19, with permission.)

a rise in hCG titer from an intercurrent pregnancy as evidence of choriocarcinoma. There has been some suspicion for many years that the female sex steroids in hormonal contraceptives may promote the persistence of molar trophoblast and should therefore not be used (5). Stone et al. (20) reported the first direct data on this important aspect (Table 6), and their results support this suspicion. More recently, Berkowitz et al. (3) published a negative report. We have used hormonal contraceptives for all our patients, but during the first half of the 1970's, intramuscular medroxyprogesterone acetate (Depo-Provera®) was used. In the second half of the 1970's, estrogen-progestin oral contraceptives were prescribed (8). Although a nonhormonal contraceptive treatment arm is lacking in our study, the patients receiving the estrogen had a lower but not statistically significant incidence of postmolar trophoblastic disease than the progestin group, suggesting that the estrogen cannot be primarily responsible for increasing the incidence of PMTD. The experiments of Wilson et al. (27) suggest the opposite should be true, since the diagnosis of PMTD is usually based entirely on persistently elevated hCG values. Wilson and co-workers noted that in tissue culture, progestational steroids suppressed the excretion of hCG. It is our opinion that the risk of not using hormonal

TABLE 6. *Effect of hormone contraception on incidence of trophoblastic disease*

Oral contraception	Stone et al. (20)		Berkowitz et al. (3)		Eddy et al. (8)	
	N	TD (%)	N	TD (%)	N	TD (%)
Yes	64	25	58	19	71	20
No	464	9.3	42	14	32[a]	31

[a]Received intramuscular medroxyprogesterone acetate 150 mg every 2 to 3 months for contraception.
N: total number of cases of molar pregnancy, TD: trophoblastic disease.

contraceptives, namely, pregnancy, for our patients is greater than the probability that the contraceptives increase the risk for trophoblastic neoplasia.

REPEAT CURETTAGE

It has been a long-standing practice for many clinicians to routinely curet the uterus a week or so after a molar pregnancy has been evacuated. The purpose of the second curettage was to assure complete evacuation of the molar tissue, since it was accepted that persistent elevation in titers was sometimes, if not usually, caused by retained tissue accessible to the curet. Others reserved repeat curettage for postmolar patients with persistent titers, an enlarged uterus, or bleeding.

It has been our policy to follow vacuum curettage with a gentle mechanical curettage, submitting the specimens separately for microscopic study. We have noted that the second specimen seldom had any molar tissue, even from cases that manifested persistent elevation of the hCG titers. Furthermore, we have observed that patients subsequently curetted for bleeding usually had little tissue, whether the uterus was large or not. Consequently, we undertook a program of curetting all patients whose titer plateaued or rose following molar pregnancy. Of 11 patients managed in this way, only 2 had any significant molar tissue recovered. Both had a subsequent sustained decrease in the hCG titer to normal, and neither patient had her molar pregnancy terminated at our hospital. The remaining 9 cases, all evacuated at our institution, had no titer drop or only a transient decline. Each patient went into remission with chemotherapy.

Based on our experience and understanding of the problem, routine curettage seems unnecessary. The major indication would be clinically significant bleeding. In these cases, chemotherapy also should be initiated to prevent progression of the tumor, with perforation or hemorrhage necessitating a hysterectomy.

PROPHYLACTIC CHEMOTHERAPY

Although the administration of a single course of actinomycin D or methotrexate can in most cases eradicate invasive molar tissue and, perhaps, choriocarcinoma coexistent with molar pregnancy, it does not prevent these complications but rather reduces the apparent frequency with which they occur. What is prevented is the clinical manifestation of their presence. Today, no one would recommend prophylactic chemotherapy for all cases of molar pregnancy, since certain features of molar pregnancy have been identified (7,9,14) characterizing cases most likely to be complicated by proliferative, invasive lesions (Table 7). These features, usually recognizable at the time of diagnosis, are present in about 40% of all cases of molar pregnancy. However, we do not recommend preemptive chemotherapy in these cases either, because only one-half of them will prove to need treatment if the hCG regression curve is used to identify the cases with PMTD. Chemotherapy may be administered to the patient with a high-risk molar pregnancy whose progress cannot be followed after evacuation; but this is an unusual situation even among our indigent patients.

INDICATIONS FOR TREATMENT OF PMTD

The diagnosis of PMTD based on an abnormal hCG regression curve is quite reliable, but not all patients with this diagnosis will need treatment. Figure 3 shows a typical normal hCG regression curve; each weekly titer is less than the upper limits of the normal range. An occasional patient will have elevated hCG titers, which, however, drop progressively to normal (Fig. 4). These cases certainly need no therapeutic intervention. In Fig. 5, an early plateau has occurred in the range of 3,000 to 4,000 mIU/ml. It was sustained for 4 weeks despite an elective curettage. Chemotherapy quickly induced a titer remission. For the woman with nonmetastatic PMTD, hysterectomy is the treatment of choice, provided the patient has completed her family. An example of this is depicted in Fig. 6. The patient had a rapidly rising titer over a 3-week period. Hysterectomy was followed by a precipitous decline in the hCG serum values to normal (<1 mIU/ml).

As soon as a plateau or rise occurs based on serial hCG values or a single elevated titer occurs without reference levels, a chest X ray should be obtained. If it is negative and the plateau is in the range of 500 mIU/ml or less, we continue to monitor the patient expectantly for several weeks. With titers higher than 500 mIU/ml or if lung metastases are present, brain and liver scans are obtained and chemotherapy instituted. Other than the presence of metastases or abnormal titers, the only indication for instituting therapy for PMTD is major uterine bleeding. Such patients, however, almost invariably have abnormal hCG regression curves.

TABLE 7. *Features of molar pregnancy associated with high risk for trophoblastic disease*

Uterus large for dates
Theca-lutein cysts
Preevacuation serum hCG titer > 100,000 mIU/ml
Maternal age > 40
Prior molar pregnancy or trophoblastic tumor
Toxemia, hyperthyroidism

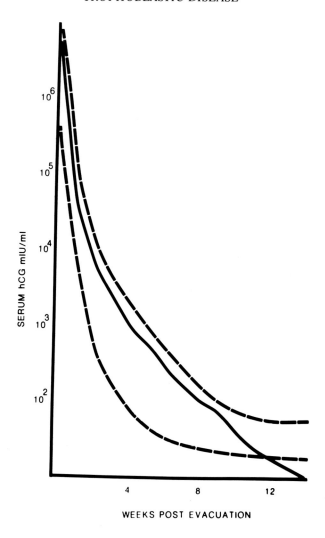

SERUM hCG mIU/ml

WEEKS POST EVACUATION

FIG. 3. Patient M. N. Molar pregnancy evacuated February 14, 1977. Weekly serum hCG values exhibit progressive drop to undetectable levels at 13 weeks. All values within 95% confidence range of normal. Patient does not have invasive mole or choriocarcinoma.

TREATMENT REGIMENS FOR NONMETASTATIC PMTD

The standard 5-day methotrexate or actinomycin D regimens are listed in Table 8. They are highly effective but have the disadvantages of frequent toxicity and frequent visits to the doctor. Because the chemotherapy of trophoblastic tumors is very schedule-dependent, these drug courses are usually repeated about every 2 weeks. This means that the patient will be going to the physician's office 5 out of every 10 working days. If the patient returns on day 8 for a weekly hCG titer and blood count, then a 6th day of travel is required. The toxicity is generally tolerable,

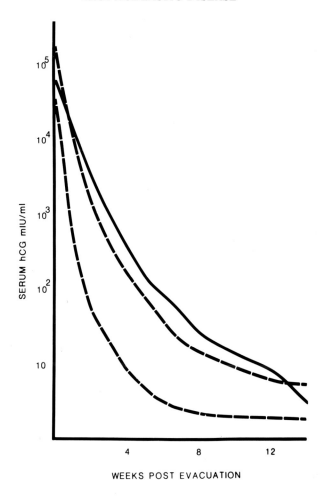

FIG. 4. Patient L. S. Atypical postmolar serum hCG regression. Each weekly titer shows progressive decline to nondetectable level at 14 weeks. However, all values slightly above 95% confidence limits until week 13. Patient does not have invasive mole or choriocarcinoma.

although the methotrexate tends to accumulate, causing somewhat unpredictable problems with stomatitis and bone-marrow depression. The 10-µg/kg dose of actinomycin D produces some hair loss, serious bone-marrow depression, and dermatitis; nausea with or without vomiting occurs daily in most patients during the week of treatment. For the past 2 years, we have used a pulse dose of actinomycin D once every 2 weeks. This is extremely convenient for the patient, since it requires only 1 office visit each treatment course. If given on a Friday afternoon, the patient has the weekend to recover from the gastrointestinal side effects.

The alternating methotrexate-citrovorum factor 8-day regimen, which has the great advantage of very little toxicity, has been used by Bagshawe and Begent (1)

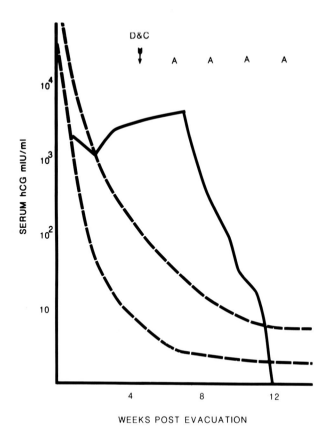

WEEKS POST EVACUATION

FIG. 5. Patient B. A. Regression curve exhibits typical early departure from normal indicating presence of proliferating trophoblastic tissue, i.e., invasive mole or choriocarcinoma. hCG titer continued to rise despite repeat uterine curettage at 4.5 weeks postevacuation. Logarithmic fall in titer after initiation of chemotherapy (actinomycin D 5-day regimen) is usual. Patient received one course after first negative titer (<1.0 mIU/ml).

and by Goldstein (2). Unfortunately, it requires frequent office visits or hospitalization over the weekend. Patient compliance is an absolute necessity to ensure that the patient is "rescued" with citrovorum factor every other day.

TREATMENT REGIMENS FOR METASTATIC TROPHOBLASTIC DISEASE

The success of single-agent and combination drug therapy for metastatic trophoblastic disease (Table 9) is one of the marvels of contemporary medicine, but it is this very success that has made so difficult the acceptance of the failures that do occur. The patients with choriocarcinoma whose prognosis is still poor today are those with brain or liver metastases. Such patients usually also have relatively long-standing disease and high titers. Whole-brain irradiation (3,000 rads over a period of 2 to 3 weeks) is very effective in preventing fatal hemorrhage and is

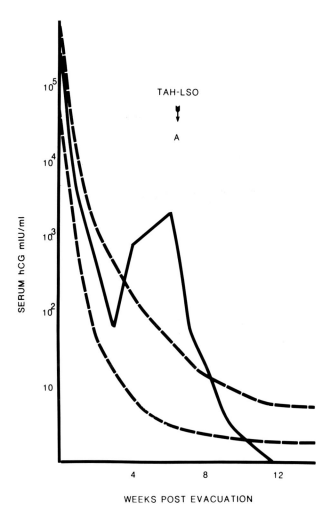

FIG. 6. Patient J. P. Following hysterectomy, serum hCG drops from 2500 mIU/ml to non-detectable levels (<1.0 mIU/ml) in 6 weeks. Hysterectomy performed during 5-day course of actinomycin D chemotherapy. We no longer employ chemotherapy to "cover" patients during surgical procedures.

probably also locally curative. None of our 9 cases have failed in the brain clinically, but 5 have died of persistent lung metastases. Whether or not liver irradiation is helpful remains to be demonstrated. Certainly it has the potential to prevent fatal hemorrhage, but it is also not well tolerated, especially in conjunction with intensive chemotherapy.

Recently, two combination drug regimens have been reported that appear to offer hope to patients failing conventional triple-drug therapy, whether the reason for failure is toxicity preventing adequate drug treatment, or actual drug resistance. Figure 7 presents the titer response in a patient incapable of tolerating methotrexate

TABLE 8. *Chemotherapy for nonmetastatic PMTD*

Standard regimens[a]	
Methotrexate	0.4 mg/kg/d. i.v. or i.m. × 5d. q. 2 weeks
Actinomycin D	10 μg/kg/d. i.v. × 5d. q. 2 weeks
Alternate regimens	
Actinomycin D[b]	1 mg/m² i.v. × 1d. q. 2 weeks
Methotrexate[c] and	1.0 mg/kg i.m., days 1, 3, 5, 7 ⎫ q. 3 weeks
Citrovorum factor	0.1 mg/kg i.m., days 2, 4, 6, 8 ⎭

[a]From Morrow and Townsend (15).
[b]From Petrilli and Morrow (17).
[c]From Berkowitz and Goldstein (2).

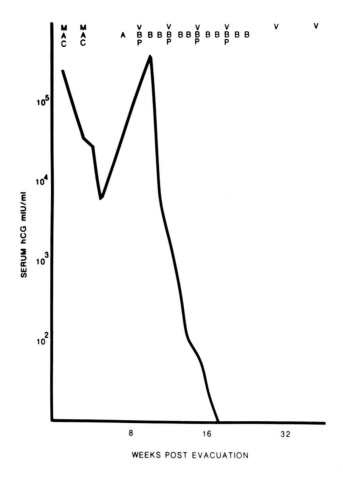

FIG. 7. Patient C. M., with high-risk metastatic choriocarcinoma. Responded well to conventional triple drug therapy (MAC) indicated by slashes at top of graph. Because of severe serositis, patient given actinomycin D only on third course. With no titer response to single agent actinomycin D patient treated with vinblastine, bleomycin, and *cis*-platinum. Titer response was precipitous, falling from 350,000 mIU/ml to nondetectable levels after only three courses (9 weeks). Patient remains in remission more than 2 years later.

TABLE 9. *Conventional combination chemotherapy for metastatic trophoblastic disease*

Drug	Regimen
Methotrexate	0.3 mg/kg/d. i.v. × 5 d.
Actinomycin D	8 μg/kg/d. i.v. × 5 d.
Cyclophosphamide[a]	3 mg/kg/d. i.v. × 5 d.

[a]Leukeran 0.15 mg/kg/d. orally may be substituted for cyclophosphamide.
From Morrow and Townsend (15).

and unresponsive to actinomycin D who achieved complete remission with 4 courses of vinblastine (Velban®), bleomycin, and *cis*-platinum (Table 10), which has been reported in full elsewhere (18). Bagshawe and Begent (1) have devised a 7-drug regimen, which includes methotrexate, actinomycin D, and cyclophosphamide (Table 11). They believe it is more effective and less toxic than the conventional combined methotrexate, actinomycin D, and cyclophosphamide (MAC) regimen. It may also prove effective in cases that are known to be resistant to MAC (21).

TABLE 10. *Vinblastine, bleomycin, and cis-platinum regimen for choriocarcinoma*

Vinblastine	9 mg/m² i.v., day 1
Bleomycin	20 μ/m² i.m. weekly
Cis-platinum	20 mg/m²/d. i.v., days 1–5
Repeat vinblastine and *cis*-platinum q. 3 weeks	

TABLE 11. *Bagshawe's CHAMOCA regimen*

Day	Time	Regimen	
1		Hydroxyurea	1 g q.d.s., for 24 hr
2	10:00 a.m.	Vincristine	1.0 mg/m² stat i.v.
	3:00 p.m.	Methotrexate	100 mg/m² stat i.v.
		Methotrexate	200 mg/m² 12-hr infusion i.v.
3	3:00 p.m.	Folinic acid	15 mg i.m. or p.o.
4	8:00 a.m.	Folinic acid	15 mg i.m. or p.o.
	10:00 a.m.	Cyclophosphamide	600 mg/m² i.v.
		Actinomycin D	0.5 mg i.v.
	8:00 p.m.	Folinic acid	15 mg i.m. or p.o.
5	8:00 a.m.	Folinic acid	15 mg. i.m. or p.o.
	10:00 a.m.	Actinomycin D	0.5 mg i.v.
6	10:00 a.m.	Actinomycin D	0.5 mg i.v.
7		No treatment	
8		No treatment	
9		Adriamycin[a]	30 mg/m² i.v.
		Cyclophosphamide[a]	400 mg/m² i.v.

[a]Check white blood cell count and platelets before giving.
From Bagshawe and Begent (1).

ACKNOWLEDGMENT

This work was supported in part by National Institutes of Health Grant No. 20749.

REFERENCES

1. Bagshawe, K. D., and Begent, R. H. (1981): Trophoblastic tumors: clinical features and management. In: *Gynecologic Oncology*, edited by M. Coppleson, pp. 757–772. Churchill Livingstone, London.
2. Berkowitz, R. S., and Goldstein, D. P. (1979): Methotrexate with citrovorum factor rescue for nonmetastatic gestational trophoblastic neoplasms. *Obstet. Gynecol.*, 54:725–728.
3. Berkowitz, R. S., Goldstein, D. P., Marean, A. R., and Bernstein, M. (1981): Oral contraceptives and postmolar trophoblastic disease. *Obstet. Gynecol.*, 58:474–477.
4. Brewer, J. I., Eckman, T. R., Dolkart, R. E., Torok, E. E., and Webster, A. (1971): Gestational trophoblastic disease: A comparative study of the results of therapy in patients with invasive mole and with choriocarcinoma. *Am. J. Obstet. Gynecol.*, 109:335–340.
5. Brewer, J. I., Halpern, B., and Torok, E. E. (1979): Gestational trophoblastic disease: Selected clinical aspects and chorionic gonadotropin test methods pp. 1–43. In: *Current Problems in Cancer.* Year Book Medical Publishers, Chicago.
6. Cotton, D. B., Bernstein, S. G., Read, J. A., Benedetti, T. I., D'Ablaing, G., Miller, F. C., and Morrow, C. P. (1980): Hemodynamic observations in evacuation of molar pregnancy. *Am. J. Obstet. Gynecol.*, 138:6–10.
7. Curry, S. L., Hammond, C. B., Tyrey, L., Creasman, W. T., and Parker, R. T. (1975): Hydatidiform mole: Diagnosis, management and long-term followup. *Obstet. Gynecol.*, 45:1–8.
8. Eddy, G. L., Schlaerth, J. B., Nalick, R. H., Nakamura, R. M., and Morrow, C. P. (1981): Influence of contraceptive methods on the development of post-molar trophoblastic disease. *Annual Meeting of the American College of Obstetricians and Gynecologists*. Las Vegas, Nevada.
9. Goldstein, D. P., Berkowitz, R. S., and Cohen, S. M. (1979): The current management of molar pregnancy pp. 1–41. In: *Current Problems in Obstetrics and Gynecology.* Year Book Medical Publishers, Chicago.
10. Hatch, K. D., Shingleton, H. M., Austin, J. M., Boots, L. R., Younger, B., and Soong, S. J. (1978): Southern Regional Trophoblastic Disease Center, 1972–1977. *South. Med. J.*, 71:1334–1340.
11. Hohe, P. T., Cochrane, C. R., Gmelich, J. T., and Austin, J. A. (1971): Coexistent trophoblastic tumor and viable pregnancy. *Obstet. Gynecol.*, 38:899–904.
12. Kajii, T., and Ohama, K. (1977): Androgenetic origin of hydatidiform mole. *Nature*, 268:633–634.
13. Kohorn, E. I. (1982): Hydatidiform mole and gestational trophoblastic disease in Southern Connecticut. *Obstet. Gynecol.*, 59:78–84.
14. Morrow, C. P., Kletzky, O. A., DiSaia, P. J., Townsend, D. E., Mishell, D. R., and Nakamura, R. M. (1977): Clinical and laboratory correlates of molar pregnancy and trophoblastic disease. *Am. J. Obstet. Gynecol.*, 128:424–429.
15. Morrow, C. P., and Townsend, D. E. (1981): *Synopsis of Gynecologic Oncology*, 2nd ed. John Wiley & Sons, New York.
16. Pattillo, R. A., Sasaki, S., Katayama, K. P., Roesler, M., and Mattingly, R. F. (1981): Genesis of 46,XY hydatidiform mole. *Am. J. Obstet. Gynecol.*, 141:104–106.
17. Petrilli, E. S., and Morrow, C. P. (1980): Actinomycin D toxicity in the treatment of trophoblastic disease. *Gynecol. Oncol.*, 9:18–22.
18. Schlaerth, J. B., Morrow, C. P., and DePetrillo, A. D. (1980): Sustained remission of choriocarcinoma with cis-platinum, vinblastine, and bleomycin after failure of conventional drug therapy. *Am. J. Obstet. Gynecol.*, 136:983–985.
19. Schlaerth, J. B., Morrow, C. P., Kletzky, O. A., Nalick, R. H., and D'Ablaing, G. (1981): Prognostic characteristics of serum human chorionic gonadotropin titer regression following molar pregnancy. *Obstet. Gynecol.*, 58:478–482.
20. Stone, M., Dent, J., Kardana, A., and Bagshawe, K. D. (1976): Relationship of oral contraception to development of trophoblastic tumour after evacuation of a hydatidiform mole. *Br. J. Obstet. Gynaecol.*, 83:913–916.

21. Surwit, E. A., Suciu, T. N., Schmidt, H. J., and Hammond, C. B. (1979): A new combination chemotherapy for resistant trophoblastic disease. *Gynecol. Oncol.*, 8:110–118.
22. Szulman, A. E., and Surti, U. (1978): The syndromes of hydatidiform mole: Cytogenetic and morphologic correlations. *Am. J. Obstet. Gynecol.*,131:665–671.
23. Szulman, A. E., Surti, U., and Berman, M. (1978): Patient with partial mole requiring chemotherapy. *Lancet*, 2:1099.
24. Szulman, A. E., Ma, H. K., Wong, L. C., and Hsu, C. (1981): Residual trophoblastic disease in association with partial hydatidiform mole. *Obstet. Gynecol.*, 57:392–394.
25. Twiggs, L. B., Morrow, C. P., and Schlaerth, J. B. (1979): Acute pulmonary complications of molar pregnancy. *Am. J. Obstet. Gynecol.*, 135:189–194.
26. Vassilakos, P., Riotton, G., and Kajii, T. (1977): Hydatidiform mole: Two entities. *Am. J. Obstet. Gynecol.*, 127:167–170.
27. Wilson, E. A., Jawad, M. J., and Dickson, L. R. (1980): Suppression of human chorionic gonadotropin by progestational steroids. *Am. J. Obstet. Gynecol.*, 138:708–713.

Recent Clinical Developments in Gynecologic Oncology, edited by C. Paul Morrow, et al. Raven Press, New York © 1983.

Atypical Hyperplasia and Adenocarcinoma of the Endometrium

H. Fox

Department of Pathology, Stopford Building, University of Manchester, Manchester M13 9PT, England

The question of endometrial hyperplasia and its relationship to and differentiation from endometrial adenocarcinoma may appear at first glance to be a relatively simple one. This unfortunately is not the case, partly because it is in fact not a simple question and partly because its complexity has been compounded by variations in terminology and definitions, by differences in conceptual attitudes, and by the inability among pathologists to agree on the criteria for distinguishing between hyperplasia and adenocarcinoma. Indeed, the situation has become so confused that it is now almost traditional for anyone reviewing this topic to begin their discussion with a table in which the various diagnostic labels attached by different authorities to a particular histological type of hyperplasia are detailed, compared, and contrasted (18,20). This is usually followed by a second comparative table, in which the varying criteria suggested by different authors for distinguishing hyperplasia and adenocarcinoma are listed. Such tables give the reviewer a feeling of academic satisfaction and completeness but tend to induce in those forced to peruse them a curious mixture of tedium and confusion.

In the discussion in this chapter, these almost ritualistic preambles are largely, although not entirely, dispensed with, and a personal viewpoint is presented. It is not by any means claimed that the terminology and definitions used here are any better or any more likely to be correct than those used in other accounts of endometrial hyperplasia, but they do appear to be applicable in practice without excessive confusion and are relatively free of semantic and conceptual contradictions.

CLASSIFICATION OF ENDOMETRIAL HYPERPLASIA

Endometrial hyperplasia is not a single entity, and to use this term without any qualifying adjective not only denies the existence of a variety of hyperplastic conditions of the endometrium but also conceals their independent and vastly different relationships to the subsequent development of endometrial adenocarcinoma.

Four forms of endometrial hyperplasia can be recognized histologically:

1. Cystic glandular hyperplasia.
2. Adenomatoid hyperplasia.

3. Glandular hyperplasia with architectural atypia.
4. Glandular hyperplasia with cytological atypia.

The fourth form of hyperplasia is synonymous with the term "atypical hyperplasia," and there is no real objection to the use of this term except that it is also often applied to glandular hyperplasia with architectural atypia, an abnormality that is possibly of much lesser importance. A notable omission from this classification is the term "adenomatous hyperplasia," a form of nomenclature that has not only been used indiscriminately but also is indefensible in both semantic and conceptual respects, since a lesion cannot be both neoplastic and hyperplastic at the same time. The term "adenomatoid hyperplasia," on the other hand, is acceptable, since it is quite possible for a hyperplastic condition to resemble a tumor; however, this diagnostic label is restricted to an uncommon but specific form of endometrial hyperplasia and is not used as a synonym for "adenomatous hyperplasia."

PATHOLOGY OF ENDOMETRIAL HYPERPLASIA

Cystic Glandular Hyperplasia

Cystic glandular hyperplasia (Fig. 1) involves the entire endometrium, which is thickened and polypoid and often is characterized by a velvety appearance; tiny cysts may be seen even with the naked eye. The myometrium is also usually hypertrophied, and the uterus, bulky. Histologically, there is diffuse involvement of the endometrium, and the distinction between the functional and basal zones is lost. The glands are characterized by their marked variability in size—some being

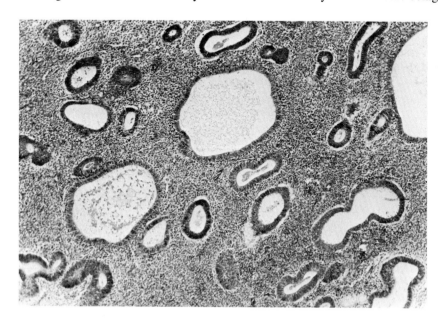

FIG. 1. Cystic glandular hyperplasia of endometrium (H. & E. ×40).

unduly large, others being normal, and still others being unusually small; they do, however, retain their regular, smooth, and rounded outlines. The glandular epithelium is formed of plump, regular columnar cells, which stain darkly and have central round nuclei. There is often a minor degree of multilayering. However, there is no loss of polarity, and cellular atypia is not seen. Mitotic figures may be common or sparse but are invariably of normal form. The ratio of stroma to glands is normal, since the stroma shares in the hyperplastic process and usually appears markedly cellular.

Adenomatoid Hyperplasia

Adenomatoid hyperplasia (Fig. 2) is a rare lesion and invariably focal in nature. It is characterized by a simple excess of glands of normal shape and approximately normal size, with a marked reduction in the intervening stroma. There is no cellular atypia, and the overall appearance differs from that of a normal proliferative endometrium only by the abundance of glands and the striking reduction, although never the complete absence, of intervening stroma.

Glandular Hyperplasia with Architectural Atypia

Glandular hyperplasia with architectural atypia (Fig. 3) is restricted to the glandular component of the endometrium and is commonly focal rather than diffuse. The glands, although variable in size, are often rather larger than normal and are more numerous, the intervening stroma being reduced. There is an abnormal pattern of glandular growth, with outpouchings, or buddings, of the glandular epithelium

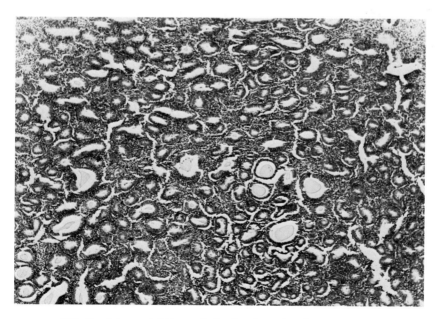

FIG. 2. Adenomatoid hyperplasia of endometrium (H. & E. ×40).

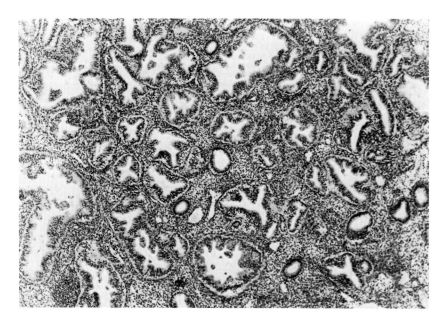

FIG. 3. Glandular hyperplasia of endometrium with architectural atypia (H. & E. ×40).

into the stroma and pseudopapillary projections of epithelium into the glandular lumen. Often the glands appear elongated, and multiple outpouchings into the stroma may impart a serrated appearance, which can be confused with that seen in a normal late secretory endometrium. The glands are lined by regular, darkly staining, cuboid cells with rounded central nuclei. There is no cellular or nuclear atypia and little stratification. Mitotic figures may be present and are of normal form.

Glandular Hyperplasia with Cellular Atypia

Glandular hyperplasia with cellular atypia (Figs. 4 and 5) is also restricted to the endometrial glands and always appears to be focal in nature, often sharply so. However, sometimes it is multifocal, and this may give a false impression of diffuse involvement, which is dispelled by careful topographic study. Such a study reveals that the foci of glands with cellular atypia are always separated from each other either by normal glands or by glands showing another variety of endometrial hyperplasia. In the affected areas of the endometrium, there is a marked reduction in stroma, and the glands either assume a "back-to-back" appearance or are separated from each other only by narrow bands of stroma. The glands may have an appearance similar to that seen in an architectural atypia but are often markedly irregular in shape and size, showing a degree of generalized irregularity and deformity that goes beyond that explicable simply in terms of multiple budding or tufting. The

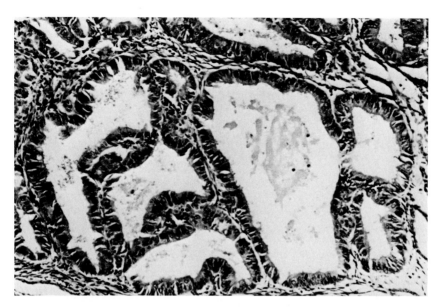

FIG. 4. Glandular hyperplasia of endometrium with cellular atypia (H. & E. ×85).

cells lining the glands show varying degrees of cellular and nuclear atypia, such as nuclear crowding, multilayering, intraluminal tufting, and mitotic activity. However, the nuclei are usually ovoid and, despite the epithelial multilayering, commonly preserve their polarity; their nucleoli are generally small, and all mitotic figures present are of normal form. The intraluminal epithelial tufts may appear to fuse with each other to give a cribiform appearance to the glands, but these apparent "bridges" retain a stromal support. The cytoplasm is usually relatively scanty and amphophilic, but in some instances, usually those with the most severe cellular atypia, it can be abundant and markedly eosinophilic.

Glandular hyperplasia with cellular atypia is commonly classified as mild, moderate, or severe. However, these terms not only represent subjective and arbitrary subdivisions of a continuous spectrum of abnormality but fail to take into account that the degree of cellular and nuclear atypia may vary not only from one area to another but even within the same gland.

INTERRELATIONSHIPS OF VARIOUS FORMS
OF ENDOMETRIAL HYPERPLASIA

Although each form of endometrial hyperplasia has been described and can exist separately and in isolation, it is not uncommon to encounter various types of hyperplasia coexisting in the same endometrium. Cystic glandular hyperplasia is

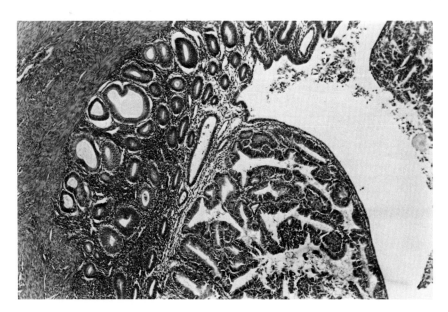

FIG. 5. Focus of glandular hyperplasia with both architectural and cellular atypia in otherwise normal endometrium. There is sharp distinction between normal and hyperplastic glands (H. & E. ×40).

frequently found in pure form but is not uncommonly seen in combination with glandular hyperplasia with architectural atypia, glandular hyperplasia with cellular atypia, or both. A pure glandular hyperplasia with architectural atypia is not uncommon, but there is often an accompanying cystic glandular hyperplasia or glandular hyperplasia with cellular atypia. It is relatively uncommon to encounter glandular hyperplasia with cellular atypia in isolated form, although it is certainly sometimes seen in the setting of an otherwise normal or even atrophic endometrium; frequently, there is an associated glandular hyperplasia with architectural atypia and/or a cystic glandular hyperplasia. The only exception to this general rule of frequent coexistence is adenomatoid hyperplasia, which always appears to develop in an otherwise normal endometrium.

These somewhat complex interrelationships may suggest that the various forms of hyperplasia are different morphological expressions of a common basic abnormality of growth or that they form a continuous spectrum. In fact, there is no evidence that cystic glandular hyperplasia is a precursor of or evolves into a purely glandular type of hyperplasia, since transitional forms between the two conditions are not seen, even when both are present in the same endometrium. Indeed, there is often a very distinct and clear boundary between the two abnormal patterns. There is also no evidence that adenomatoid hyperplasia is related in any way to cystic glandular hyperplasia or to the various forms of glandular hyperplasia with atypia. On the other hand, glandular hyperplasia with architectural atypia often does appear to evolve into glandular hyperplasia with cellular atypia, and transitional stages between the two varieties are commonly seen. What is not known is whether the form with architectural atypia commonly or even usually evolves into a glandular hyperplasia with cellular atypia or is indeed a necessary and inevitable precursor stage.

ETIOLOGY AND PATHOGENESIS OF ENDOMETRIAL HYPERPLASIA

It is generally accepted that all forms of endometrial hyperplasia, with the possible exception of adenomatoid hyperplasia, can be caused by and indeed are usually the result of prolonged unopposed estrogenic stimulation of the endometrium, whether this be the result of a series of anovulatory cycles, an estrogenic ovarian tumor, or the administration of exogenous estrogens. It is almost certainly the case that virtually all women whose endometrium is subjected to prolonged estrogenic stimulation will eventually develop some degree of cystic glandular hyperplasia and that this form of hyperplasia does not occur except under conditions of sustained estrogen drive. This, together with the diffuse involvement of glands, stroma, and myometrium, suggests that this type of hyperplasia is the expected, virtually physiological, response to an abnormal degree of estrogenic stimulation; in other words, it is the normal response to an abnormal hormonal environment.

Glandular hyperplasia with atypia, either architectural or cellular, also often develops against a background of prolonged estrogenic stimulation and, in such cases, usually coexists with a cystic glandular hyperplasia. However, glandular hyperplasia with atypia is always focal rather than diffuse and can develop when there are no reasons to suspect an endocrinological abnormality, being, as already noted, sometimes found as a localized lesion in an otherwise normal, or atrophic, endometrium. Therefore, it seems reasonable to suggest that these forms of hyperplasia represent a local tissue abnormality, which can be independent of estrogenic stimulation but is more commonly estrogen induced. The implication of this is that glandular hyperplasia with atypia is biologically fundamentally different from cystic glandular hyperplasia. Indeed, it is possible that the lesion called glandular hyperplasia with atypia is not a true hyperplasia but basically represents a neoplastic reaction, a point considered in greater detail later.

Adenomatoid hyperplasia is rare but usually occurs focally in an otherwise normal endometrium, and therefore there are no grounds for believing that it is related to estrogenic stimulation. The appearance of the lesion suggests strongly that far from being an adenomatoid lesion, it is a true adenoma of the endometrium. It has always appeared strange that nonmalignant neoplasms of the endometrium do not appear to exist, and this deficiency would be repaired by the acceptance of adenomatoid hyperplasia as a benign tumor.

NATURE OF ENDOMETRIAL ADENOCARCINOMA *IN SITU*

Before discussing the distinction between glandular hyperplasia with marked cellular atypia and adenocarcinoma, it is necessary to consider precisely what is meant in this particular context by adenocarcinoma. It is perfectly clear that an adenocarcinoma that is invading the myometrium is a true malignant neoplasm, but there has been and still is considerable controversy regarding the meaning of carcinoma *in situ* of the endometrium (5,7). The term "endometrial adenocarcinoma *in situ*" has been used in three quite different ways, although this is not always clear in descriptions of endometrial pathology, some authors using the same term in two or more different senses in the same account. Some equate endometrial adenocarcinoma *in situ* with glandular hyperplasia showing marked cellular atypia, while others, although drawing a distinction between these two entities, do not always elaborate as to whether they consider an *in situ* adenocarcinoma to be one that is not invading the endometrial stroma or one that is not invading the myometrium. An adenocarcinoma *in situ* is by definition a noninvasive lesion, and therefore a true adenocarcinoma *in situ* of the endometrium is one in which the glands have undergone neoplastic change but in which there is no invasion of the endometrial stroma. However, it is doubtful if an adenocarcinoma of this type exists, or if it could be recognized even if it did exist. Therefore, some form of nomenclature has to be found to describe an invasive adenocarcinoma that is confined to the endometrium. The term "stage 0 carcinoma" has been applied to a lesion of this type (7), but this appears to use a clinical staging to describe a histological finding. The term "focal adenocarcinoma" is inappropriate for a tumor that is invading the myometrium may also be focal, while "early adenocarcinoma" is too imprecise. The term "intraendometrial adenocarcinoma" has much to recommend it, while, as will be considered later, a case can be made for classifying such a lesion as "intraendometrial neoplasia."

DISTINCTION BETWEEN HYPERPLASIA AND ADENOCARCINOMA

The need to differentiate between a glandular hyperplasia with severe cellular atypia and a well-differentiated (grade 1) adenocarcinoma is one of the pathologist's most difficult tasks. In a hysterectomy specimen, this task is, of course, simpler, because if there is definite myometrial invasion, then the lesion is, irrespective of morphological niceties, an adenocarcinoma. If there is no invasion of the myometrium, then no practical necessity arises for differentiating the two conditions, insofar as they both have the same excellent prognosis and are both treated by the therapeutic measure that has already been performed. The difficulty is therefore encountered in its most acute form in curettage material. Suggested criteria indicating that the glands are neoplastic rather than hyperplastic include (8,14,17,18) the formation of intraglandular bridges without stromal support, the presence of nuclear debris and polymorphs within glandular lumina, the stratification of cells to form a "glands within glands" pattern, the loss of nuclear polarity, the presence of marked nuclear irregularity, the rounding of the nuclei, the prominence of the nucleoli, the presence of pale eosinophilic cytoplasm, numerous mitotic figures, or abnormal mitotic figures, the complete absence of stroma between glands, and the piling up of cells into random sheets and masses. Suggested features indicating stromal invasion and therefore implying the malignant nature of the glands include fibrosis of the stroma between the glands, focal stromal necrosis, and stromal accumulation of histiocytes.

Those who have attempted to compile such a list of distinguishing characteristics have often failed to indicate whether they are drawing a distinction between hyperplasia and intraendometrial adenocarcinoma or between hyperplasia and an adenocarcinoma that is truly invasive insofar as it is penetrating the myometrium. Only Hendrickson and Kempson (8) have clearly defined their aims and have indicated that they are attempting to differentiate between hyperplasia and the best-differentiated adenocarcinomas that have been observed to behave biologically as carcinomas, i.e., adenocarcinomas that have invaded the myometrium. If this is taken as the acceptable aim, then a true guide to achieving it can only be gained by a retrospective analysis of the distinguishing features seen in curettage specimens from patients in whom a subsequent hysterectomy revealed an adenocarcinoma invading the myometrium. If this is done, it soon becomes clear that many of the distinguishing features listed above are of dubious or minimal value in the differential diagnosis. However, a number of findings do stand out as being of real significance, such as the presence of true intraglandular epithelial bridges devoid of stromal support, the presence of polymorphs and nuclear debris within the glandular lumens and cellular anarchy. The term "cellular anarchy," perhaps requires some explanation. I would apply it to the piling up of cells with rounded, irregular nuclei and scanty cytoplasm into sheets and masses, which is sometimes seen focally within a gland that appears otherwise to have a fairly regular epithelium. A further valid differentiating point is the presence of abnormal mitotic figures; unfortunately, these are rarely seen. It is, of course, virtually impossible to determine which of these features is the most important, although I would regard cellular anarchy as the most valuable. Should adenocarcinoma be diagnosed if only one of these features is present, or should one insist on at least two of these criteria of malignancy being met? This is theoretically a difficult question but one that in practice is rarely posed, since it is almost unknown to encounter a case in which the general appearance of hyperplasia is modified by the presence of only one of these morphological abnormalities.

These features, if seen in a curettage specimen, therefore suggest that an invasive adenocarcinoma is present. However, the question remains whether or not it is possible to distinguish between a glandular hyperplasia with marked cellular atypia and an intraendometrial adenocarcinoma. This is only possible if definite evidence of stromal invasion is seen, and suggestive features certainly do include stromal fibrosis and necrosis. Unfortunately, these changes are rarely present, and it therefore commonly becomes a matter of opinion rather than of fact whether one is dealing with a hyperplastic state or an intraendometrial adenocarcinoma.

RISK OF DEVELOPMENT OF ADENOCARCINOMA IN ENDOMETRIAL HYPERPLASIA

Attempts to establish the relationship, if any, between the presence of endometrial hyperplasia and the subsequent development of an adenocarcinoma have usually involved prospective follow-up of cases of endometrial hyperplasia, retrospective analyses of curettings from women who have later developed an endometrial adenocarcinoma, and studies of the nonneoplastic portion of the endometrium in which an adenocarcinoma is present (1,2,4,6,9,11–13,15,16,19). The number of prospective studies has been small, and in many, the true natural history of the disease has been obscured by the administration of various forms of therapy, including irradiation, to a high proportion of the patients. Retrospective analyses, of course, give a highly biased and an unduly gloomy view of the risk of adenocarcinoma in hyperplastic conditions insofar as they selectively focus on women with preceding hyperplasia and with clinical symptoms. The study of the nonneoplastic portion of an endometrium in which an adenocarcinoma is present can provide valuable information if the nonneoplastic endometrium is atrophic. However, if it is hyperplastic, then it can be very difficult to ascertain if it shows a glandular hyperplasia with severe cellular atypia or an intraendometrial adenocarcinoma.

Quite apart from the methodological difficulties that have beset attempts to establish the true risk of endometrial adenocarcinoma in endometrial hyperplasia, the greatest problems encountered in attempting to probe this relationship between the two conditions are the terminological morass, which often leaves one with a complete uncertainty about the type of hyperplasia being discussed, and the common failure to state whether the diagnosis of adenocarcinoma is based on the presence of myometrial invasion or not.

Within the obviously marked limitations imposed by these drawbacks, a few conclusions emerge with some degree of clarity. The first conclusion is that women with a cystic glandular hyperplasia of the endometrium have only a marginally increased risk of developing an invasive endometrial adenocarcinoma (11,16). Indeed, it is doubtful that a pure cystic glandular hyperplasia of the endometrium ever evolves into an adenocarcinoma, cases of frank neoplasia usually being a consequence of focal glandular hyperplasia with atypia occurring in the setting of a cystic glandular hyperplasia. It is also clear that glandular hyperplasia with cellular atypia can and does progress to an adenocarcinoma, but there are few reliable guidelines for assessing the degree of risk of such cases. The quoted incidence of the development of endometrial adenocarcinoma in cases of glandular hyperplasia with cellular atypia has varied enormously. An educated guess would be that approximately 10% of women with this form of endometrial hyperplasia will eventually develop an adenocarcinoma (3); however, it must be emphasized that this is a guess rather than a hard or proven fact.

There still remains the question of the malignant potential of glandular hyperplasia with architectural but not cellular atypia. No figures are available permitting an assessment. Again, only a guess can be made that it is probable that there is a very low risk of the eventual development of an adenocarcinoma in such cases.

NATURE OF RELATIONSHIP BETWEEN ENDOMETRIAL HYPERPLASIA AND ADENOCARCINOMA

A consideration of a number of observations leads one to look at the nature and terminology of glandular hyperplasia in a new light:

1. Cystic glandular hyperplasia is a truly hyperplastic process that involves not only the endometrial glands but also the stroma and myometrium. It does not carry any significant risk of evolving into an adenocarcinoma.

2. Glandular hyperplasia with cellular atypia involves only the endometrial glands, and these only focally. It can be provoked by estrogenic stimulation but can also arise spontaneously.

3. Glandular hyperplasia with cellular atypia can evolve into an endometrial adenocarcinoma but can also either remain stationary or regress. The incidence of overt malignant change is unknown, but such change is certainly not inevitable and probably not very common.

4. Morphologically, glandular hyperplasia with severe cellular atypia merges almost imperceptibly into intraendometrial adenocarcinoma. An intraendometrial adenocarcinoma can probably remain confined to the endometrium for a considerable length of time and does not always progress to an invasive adenocarcinoma.

Consideration of these points leads ineluctably to a comparison with cervical intraepithelial neoplasia. Glandular hyperplasia with cellular atypia clearly differs from a true endometrial hyperplasia. It is perfectly possible that it is, just as is the case with cervical intraepithelial neoplasia, a neoplastic process from the outset, albeit one that is capable of spontaneous arrest or reversal. Therefore, it seems reasonable to suggest that we reconsider the nomenclature of both glandular hyperplasia with cellular atypia and intraendometrial adenocarcinoma and regard glandular hyperplasia with mild cellular atypia as intraendometrial neoplasia (IEN) grade 1, cases with moderate atypia as IEN grade 2, and cases with both glandular hyperplasia with severe cellular atypia and intraendometrial adenocarcinoma as IEN grade 3. Cases that evolve into an invasive adenocarcinoma often show only very superficial myometrial invasion, and such cases can be compared to a microinvasive carcinoma of the cervix.

This concept of IEN has been proposed before (15) and has not been received with any great enthusiasm. Indeed, the theme of a continuous spectrum of abnormality has been challenged by the observation that at the ultrastructural level the cells in a glandular hyperplasia with severe cellular atypia differ from those in an intraendometrial adenocarcinoma by showing a lack of estrogen-induced morphological features, such as microvilli and cilia (3). However, this has not been everyone's experience (10) and, even if true, would not be an impregnable barrier to the concept of a continuous process. All the disadvantages that have been claimed for the use of the term "cervical intraepithelial neoplasia" also apply with equal force to the use of the term "intraendometrial neoplasia"; they include the application of the term "neoplasia" to a nonmalignant process, the risk of overtreatment of relatively innocuous abnormalities, and the possible psychological ill effects of a diagnosis of neoplastic disease. On the other hand, it could be argued that these disadvantages are outweighed by the possible benefits of a more realistic view of the basic biological nature of the process and by the hope that this may eventually lead to a more rational and planned therapeutic approach to these conditions than that which currently prevails.

REFERENCES

1. Beutler, H. K., Dockerty, M. B., and Randall, L. M. (1963): Precancerous lesions of the endometrium. *Am. J. Obstet. Gynecol.*, 86:433–443.
2. Campbell, P. E., and Barter, R. A. (1961): The significance of atypical endometrial hyperplasia. *J. Obstet. Gynaec. Br. Emp.*, 68:668–672.
3. Ferenczy, A. (1980): The ultrastructural dynamics of endometrial hyperplasia and neoplasia. In: *Advances in Clinical Cytology*, edited by L. G. Koss and D. V. Coleman, pp. 1–43. Butterworths, London.
4. Gore, H. (1973): Hyperplasia of the endometrium. In: *The Uterus*, edited by H. J. Norris, A. T. Hertig, and M. R. Abell, pp. 255–275. Williams and Wilkins, Baltimore.
5. Gore, H., and Hertig, A. T. (1966): Carcinoma in situ of the endometrium. *Am. J. Obstet. Gynecol.*, 94:134–155.
6. Greene, R. R., Roddick, J. W., Jr., and Milligan, M. (1958): Estrogens, endometrial hyperplasia and endometrial cancer. *Ann. N.Y. Acad. Sci.*, 75:586–599.
7. Gusberg, S. B., and Kaplan, A. L. (1963): Precursors of corpus cancer. IV. Adenomatous hyperplasia as stage 0 carcinoma of the endometrium. *Am. J. Obstet. Gynecol.*, 87:662–676.
8. Hendrickson, M. R., and Kempson, R. L. (1980): *Surgical Pathology of the Uterine Corpus.* W. B. Saunders, Philadelphia.
9. Hertig, A. T., and Sommers, S. C. (1949): Genesis of endometrial carcinoma. I. Study of prior biopsies. *Cancer*, 2:946–956.
10. Klemi, P. J., Grönroos, M., Rayramo, L., and Punnonen, R. (1980): Ultrastructural features of endometrial atypical adenomatous hyperplasia and adenocarcinomas and the plasma level of estrogens. *Gynecol. Oncol.*, 9:162–169.
11. McBride, J. M. (1959): Premenopausal cystic hyperplasia and endometrial carcinoma. *J. Obstet. Gynaec. Br. Emp.*, 66:288–296.
12. Ober, W. B. (1973): Adenocarcinoma of the endometrium: A pathologist's view. In: *Endometrial Carcinoma*, edited by M. G. Brush, R. W. Taylor, and D. C. Williams, pp. 73–81. William Heinemann, London.
13. Ritzmann, H. (1978): Types of endometrial hyperplasia and their relationship to carcinoma of the endometrium. In: *Endometrial Cancer*, edited by M. G. Brush, R. J. B. King, and R. W. Taylor, pp. 118–123. Balliere Tindall, London.
14. Robertson, W. B. (1981): *The Endometrium*. Butterworths, London.
15. Sherman, A. I., and Brown, S. (1979): The precursors of endometrial carcinoma. *Am. J. Obstet. Gynecol.*, 135:947–954.
16. Schröder, R. (1954): Endometrial hyperplasia in relation to genital function. *Am. J. Obstet. Gynecol.*, 68:294–309.

17. Silverberg, S. G. (1977): *Surgical Pathology of the Uterus*. John Wiley & Sons, New York.
18. Tavassoli, F., and Kraus, F. T. (1978): Endometrial lesions in uteri resected for atypical endo-metrial hyperplasia. *Am. J. Clin. Pathol.*, 70:770–779.
19. Vellios, F. (1972): Endometrial hyperplasias, precursors of endometrial carcinoma. *Pathol. Annu.*, 7:201–229.
20. Welch, W. R., and Scully, R. E. (1977): Precancerous lesions of the endometrium. *Hum. Pathol.*, 8:503–512.

Recent Clinical Developments in Gynecologic Oncology, edited by C. Paul Morrow, et al.
Raven Press, New York © 1983.

Specific Management Problems in Endometrial Carcinoma

C. Paul Morrow

Department of Obstetrics and Gynecology, University of Southern California School of Medicine, Los Angeles, California 90033

CLINICAL STAGING

The term "staging" in oncology refers to either the means of determining the extent of a malignancy or an officially designated system of classifying a malignant disease according to its known extent. In endometrial carcinoma, the official staging is based on clinical, i.e., nonoperative, data only. The limitations of clinical staging have been recognized for many years, but in the past decade, numerous studies have quantified the degree to which this method is inaccurate (2,7,13). The resultant understaging or overstaging frequently leads to corresponding undertreatment or overtreatment.

The fundamental steps in the clinical staging of endometrial carcinoma include a chest X-ray, physical examination, and fractional curettage. The salient features to be observed are listed in Table 1. Of these, the most important are usually the determination of cervical extension and lesional grade, since parametrial extension and liver or lung metastases are uncommon.

Cervical Extension

The difficulty in determining occult cervical involvement by endometrial carcinoma has long been known. (Somewhat paradoxical is the fact that when cervical involvement is overt, as occasionally happens, the diagnosis of cervical extension also can be erroneous, since the patient may have a primary cervical carcinoma with or without extension to the endometrium, a primary carcinoma of the isthmus, or concurrent endocervical and endometrial cancers.) A number of techniques have been used to determine cervical involvement other than the traditional fractional curettage. Among these are cervical punch biopsy, cone biopsy, hysterography, and cervicohysteroscopy. However, the value of detecting occult cervical extension does not appear to be sufficient to justify cone biopsy, since the yield will be low and the impact on treatment small. Cone biopsy is also probably not sufficient to

TABLE 1. *Clinical assessment of endometrial cancer patient*

Chest X-ray

Physical examination
  Supraclavicular, axillary, inguinal nodes
  Abdomen—hepatomegaly, ascites, mass
  Pelvis—suburethral metastasis, cervical or
    parametrial extension, adnexal enlargement,
    uterine size

Fractional curettage
  Endometrial curettings
  Endocervical curettings
  Tumor histology and grade

---

warrant hysterography or hysteroscopy, considering the potential these techniques have for causing vascular or transtubal spread of cancer. Studies purporting to show that such spread does not occur are too insensitive to be regarded valid. Such studies simply compare survival rates of cases having hysterography to survival rates from historical or extramural controls. It is unlikely that an increase in mortality as large as 5% could be detected in this manner.

One of the major sources of error using the fractional curettage technique is contamination of the endocervical specimen by tissue from the endometrium. A variety of maneuvers have been devised to circumvent this problem, the most common of which is the obstruction of the communication between the endometrial cavity and the endocervical canal by a gauze pledget. The incidence of false-positive curettings can be substantially reduced by adhering to the requirement that the carcinoma infiltrate the cervical stroma. This is imperative for those treatment plans using both whole-pelvis and intracavitary radiation preoperatively, which indeed would be overtreatment for most patients with grade 1 or 2 lesions not having cervical extension. After the radiation is given, the surgical specimen will seldom have residual carcinoma in the cervix. Consequently, when preoperative radiation is employed, the clinician will not appreciate the high incidence of false-positive endocervical curettings.

The Stockholm school, which has greatly influenced the treatment of endometrial carcinoma, recommended a three-fraction curettage (6). This, of course, compounds the problem of false-positive specimens, but it also recognizes that extension of the malignancy to the lower part of the corpus is significant in terms of its behavior and the patient's prognosis. Many investigators accept that extension to the isthmus has implications similar to that of cervical extension; far fewer have taken cognizance of the increased risk of extrauterine spread if the lower third of the corpus is invaded by cancer (3). Unfortunately, this does not diminish the problem of the false-positive endocervical curettage, since such tumor fragments do not necessarily originate from a site close to the cervix.

Grade

Another source of error in the clinical staging of endometrial carcinoma is the determination of the grade solely on the basis of the curettage specimen. This is an important source, since the grade is a very strong prognostic determinant. The report of Macasaet et al. (9) indicates that this error may be substantial (Table 2). In this case, the error would lead to undertreatment if preoperative irradiation is used, since much or all of the cancer tissue would disappear during the usual waiting period before hysterectomy is performed.

Adnexal Mass

The presence of an adnexal mass with endometrial carcinoma qualifies the case for stage III designation. Even when the enlargement is caused by adnexal metastases, the staging may be erroneous, since these cases are more likely to have intraperitoneal disease. Most frequently, however, the mass is a result of a separate, concomitant ovarian neoplasm. Other causes of an adnexal mass in the patient with endometrial carcinoma are tube-ovarian abscess and diverticular disease, both contraindications to radiation therapy. In the presence of an adnexal mass, surgery should be the first step in therapy.

Lymph Node Metastases

It has long been recognized that endometrial carcinoma is capable of producing lymphatic metastases, but it was generally held that the primary nodes were in the high aortic chain, and in such cases death was inevitable. This belief persisted despite considerable evidence to the contrary in the literature (10). The first systematic study of the risk for pelvic node metastasis in early endometrial carcinoma was published in 1970 by Lewis et al. (8), whose work regarding the incidence of such metastases has been confirmed by a collaborative study of the Gynecologic Oncology Group (GOG) in the United States (2). The incidence of aortic node and

TABLE 2. *Histologic grade of endometrial carcinoma at curettage and hysterectomy*

Grade at curettage	No. patients[a]	Higher grade at hysterectomy	
		No.	%
1	39	4	10.2
2	15	3	20.0
Total	54	7	13.0

[a]Thirty-eight patients had preoperative radiation therapy.
Modified from Macasaet et al. (9).

pelvic node metastases and their relationship to grade and myometrial invasion have been determined by these investigators (Tables 3 and 4).

Peritoneal Cytology

The GOG study (4) has also confirmed the findings of Dahle (5) that malignant cells often can be recovered by lavage from the pelvic peritoneum of women with endometrial carcinoma. The results are presented in Table 5. Neither the presence of retroperitoneal lymph node metastases nor positive peritoneal cytology can be detected by the conventional steps in clinical staging. These features thus account for another source of understaging and undertreatment.

OPERATIVE TUMOR ("SPILL")

There are many treatment centers that routinely use preoperative radiotherapy for endometrial carcinoma, because, unlike postoperative radiation, it has the po-

TABLE 3. *Incidence of pelvic and aortic node metastases in 222 cases of FIGO stage I endometrial carcinoma by grade of lesion*

| Histologic grade | No. cases | With metastases | |
		Pelvic node (%)	Aortic node (%)
1	93	2.2	1.1
2	88	11.4	6.8
3	41	26.8	24.4
Total	222	10.4	7.6[a]

[a]7.6% of all cases, with 10.8% of 157 cases having aortic node sampling.
Modified from Boronow et al. (2).

TABLE 4. *Incidence of pelvic and aortic node metastases in 222 cases of FIGO stage I endometrial carcinoma by depth of muscle invasion*

| Maximum invasion | No. cases | With metastases | |
		Pelvic node (%)	Aortic node (%)
None	92	2	1
Inner $\frac{1}{3}$	80	5	6
Middle $\frac{1}{3}$	17	18	6
Outer $\frac{1}{3}$	33	42	33
Total	222	10.4	7.6

Modified from Boronow et al. (2).

TABLE 5. *Incidence of positive peritoneal cytology in patients with stage I endometrial carcinoma*

Pathologic feature	No. cases	Positive cytology	
		No.	%
Grade			
1	74	8	11
2	63	15	24
3	30	3	10
Endometrium only	72	6	8
Inner ⅓ muscle invasion	60	9	15
Middle ⅓ muscle invasion	10	3	30
Outer ⅓ muscle invasion	25	8	32
Total	167	26	13.9

Modified from Creasman et al. (4).

tential for preventing operative spread of the tumor. This perception is supported by the clinical observation that vaginal apex recurrences are more frequent when endometrial carcinoma is treated by surgery alone than by surgery following radiation therapy. Although intraoperative spill is a potential occurrence with any form of cancer, there has been a special concern for it in the case of endometrial carcinoma. In addition to the cuff recurrence problem, other supporting evidence for operative spill includes reports of coexistent surface lesions of the tube or ovary, the rarity of preoperative vaginal metastases, the distal (suburethral) predilection of preoperative vaginal metastases, and the known capacity of endometrial tissue to implant (endometriosis). Nevertheless, careful examination of the evidence leads to the inescapable conclusion that operative spill is but a small factor in the local recurrence of endometrial cancer (11). The report of Truskett and Constable (12) contains, perhaps, the most convincing evidence. Truskett and Constable found that the vaginal apex recurrence rate in a group of stage I patients with no residual carcinoma after preoperative radiation to the corpus only (no cervical or vaginal sources) was the same as the recurrence rate in a group of stage I patients receiving no radiation therapy. The spill theory also does not explain why the incidence of cuff recurrences correlates with the histologic grade, degree of myometrial invasion, and extension to the cervix, all factors that are known to correlate with the risk for lymphatic invasion (11). Furthermore, preoperative and postoperative radiation are equally effective, suggesting that the adjuvant radiation is treating disease already present in the upper vaginal and paravaginal tissues. The recent GOG data (4) and the earlier study of Dahle (5) provide an alternative explanation for cuff recurrences other than spill and lymphatic invasion. The incidence of positive pelvic peritoneal cytology is similar to the reported incidence of vaginal cuff recurrence. This is a very convenient source of malignant cells for implanting in the vaginal cuff area, i.e., the operative bed.

PREOPERATIVE RADIATION

Contraindications

Those who employ preoperative radiation should be familiar with the contraindications to its use, i.e., the indications for surgery first. The most common is the presence of a stage I, grade 1 lesion, which seldom requires adjuvant therapy. Other contraindications are the presence of an adnexal mass, a history of or concurrent pelvic abscess (tube-ovarian, appendiceal, diverticular), the presence of pyometra, numerous prior abdominal surgeries, previous abdominal-perineal resection, and pelvic kidney. The patient who fears radiation, who is unable to cooperate during a prolonged treatment course, or who has had prior radiation (cervical cancer) is also not a good candidate for radiation therapy.

Radiation-Hysterectomy Interval

If a course of preoperative radiation is undertaken, it is a common practice to wait several weeks before hysterectomy is carried out. The reasons for waiting are generally as follows: (a) resolution of radiation "reaction," (b) regression of a large, carcinomatous mass lesion, and (c) eradication of the uterine cancer ("sterilization" of the uterus). The first two are presumed to facilitate the surgical procedure, while the last is thought to provide maximum if not absolute protection against intraoperative tumor spread. None of these appear to have any substantive data to support them. What seems to be of greater relevance is that delay may be deleterious, since it provides additional time for a residual viable uterine tumor (present in 25 to 50% of cases) to involve extrauterine sites. Since there is no way to identify preoperatively those cases that have total eradication of the uterine tumor, individualization of the radiation-hysterectomy time interval would not be reliable. The waiting policy is probably most unsuited to high-grade cancers, considering they are the most rapidly growing and most aggressive. The poorly differentiated tumors also appear to be the most difficult to destroy by preoperative radiation (Table 6). To avoid the problem of delay and to utilize the surgical staging data, Boronow (1) adopted a policy of preoperative intracavitary therapy followed by hysterectomy within a week.

TABLE 6. *Influence of histologic grade on*
frequency of residual endometrial
carcinoma after preoperative radiation

Histologic grade	No. patients	Residual disease	
		No.	%
1	62	29	46.8
2	22	9	40.9
3	7	6	85.7

Modified from Macasaet et al. (9).

In summary, it can be said of the radiation-hysterectomy interval that delay has no therapeutic effect, that the risk for spread persists during the waiting period, that the highest grade lesions are the most likely to persist after radiation, and that there is seldom a technical advantage to delaying surgery. Waiting is important when indicated to permit the patient to recuperate from the acute effects of radiation therapy. While the "empty" uterus has prognostic value, this does not seem to be a sufficient reason to otherwise postpone hysterectomy, which is, after all, the most important element in endometrial cancer treatment.

MANAGEMENT OF INTERNATIONAL FEDERATION OF GYNECOLOGY AND OBSTETRICS STAGES I AND II

Surgical Staging

The major benefit of surgery before radiation therapy in endometrial cancer is highly accurate surgical-pathologic staging. Our approach to surgical staging utilizes procedures other than the removal of the uterus, tubes, and ovaries. Upon entering the abdomen, about 50 cc saline is instilled into each of the following four areas: (a) the pelvis, (b) the left colic gutter, (c) the right colic gutter, and (d) over the right lobe of the liver. The saline is withdrawn and heparin added before the entire specimen is sent to the laboratory for cytologic evaluation. The four specimens can be pooled or sent separately. After the abdomen is explored with particular attention to the liver, omentum, and retroperitoneal nodes, the hysterectomy is carried out. If the lesion is poorly differentiated or if there is deep myometrial invasion or extension to the isthmus, pelvic and paraaortic lymph node dissections are performed in the absence of positive target nodes. The dissections are not meant to be therapeutic but are rather a thorough sampling of the nodes.

Adjuvant Therapy

Should the pelvic or aortic nodes be positive, then we recommend extended field radiation. Prophylactic progestins also are prescribed empirically for these patients. If the peritoneal cytology is positive and reveals grade 1 disease, progestins are prescribed in addition to pelvic radiation. For grade 2 and 3 lesions with positive cytology as the only evidence of extrauterine spread, either intraperitoneal P32 or whole-abdomen radiation therapy is administered. Again, progestins are prescribed prophylactically. Adjuvant chemotherapy, should such prove to be effective, would be an alternative approach.

Vaginal Hysterectomy

The vaginal approach to hysterectomy for endometrial carcinoma is seldom used today because it compromises surgical staging and often surgical treatment as well. Removal of the adnexa is more difficult through the vagina, exploration of the pelvis and abdomen cannot be done, the validity of transvaginal peritoneal cytology would be questionable, and node sampling cannot be carried out. Nevertheless, there are instances in which vaginal hysterectomy may be preferable to the abdominal approach: (a) in the obese, parous woman with a well-differentiated carcinoma, (b) in the woman with signficiant pelvic relaxation and grade 1 endometrial carcinoma, and (c) in the unusual case of the patient who for medical reasons may tolerate vaginal hysterectomy but not abdominal hysterectomy.

Radical Hysterectomy

Radical hysterectomy, at first glance, seems to be well suited to encompass the known spread pattern of stage I and II endometrial carcinoma. However, the patient population tends to be obese, elderly, and diabetic and to suffer from cardiovascular disease, all conditions that increase the risks of extended pelvic surgery. Even in well-selected cases, there are problems with the use of radical hysterectomy for endometrial cancer therapy. Many if not most patients would be seriously overtreated by such surgery. Identifying the patients requiring more than a simple hysterectomy for cure is not readily done preoperatively, even after the exclusion of the grade 1 cases. Furthermore, many of the patients who may benefit from radical hysterectomy and pelvic lymphadenectomy on the basis of the risk for lymphatic spread will already have extrapelvic spread, as evidenced by positive peritoneal cytology or aortic node metastases. Intensifying regional therapy in patients with extraregional metastases is not likely to be life saving.

Therefore, the role for radical hysterectomy must remain a minor one in endometrial cancer management. The most frequent indications are in (a) the cervical cancer patient who was treated by radiation therapy and later develops endometrial cancer, (b) the occasional patient who exhibits appropriate risk factors and refuses radiation therapy, (c) the patient who has a contraindication to radiation therapy, and (d) the patient with gross cervical involvement who is physically and medically suited to radical hysterectomy.

SPECIAL MANAGEMENT PROBLEMS

Postoperative Diagnosis of Endometrial Cancer

Occasionally it happens that endometrial cancer is an unexpected finding in the hysterectomy specimen. This situation usually arises after vaginal hysterectomy. If the uterus is routinely opened in the operating suite, most such problems can be avoided. Our recommendation is to reoperate to remove the adnexa and surgically stage the patient. Recent information suggests that even in stage Ia, grade 1 cases, without significant muscle invasion the adnexa will be involved in 1 to 3% of cases (occult) (2).

Medically Inoperable Patient

Severe cardiopulmonary disease is the primary reason a patient with endometrial carcinoma is medically inoperable. Obviously, clinical judgment will vary a great deal in these cases. Nevertheless, in everyone's experience there will be patients for whom the risk of anesthesia and surgery exceed the likely benefits of hysterectomy. For patients with grade 1 lesions and a temporary contraindication to general anesthesia or who are altogether unsuited to radiation therapy or surgery, high-dose progestins are the treatment of choice. All other cases are given radiation therapy. If the uterus is small, tandem and ovoid intracavitary therapy alone is used. Patients with a large uterus probably stand a better chance of cure using the Heyman packing technique (6). Whether radiation or hormonal therapy is administered, endometrial biopsy or curettage should be performed after 3 months. If a tumor is present, the contraindications to surgery must be reassessed.

The Young Woman

The diagnosis of endometrial carcinoma during the reproductive years should always be viewed with skepticism since the malignancy is uncommon and confusion with hyperplasia is frequent. The histologic distinction between atypical hyperplasia, which can be treated hormonally, and well-differentiated carcinoma, which should be treated surgically, is to some extent subjective. When preservation of fertility is a significant clinical factor, the diagnosis of well-differentiated carcinoma should be based on endometrial curettings, and consultation with a recognized authority in the field of endometrial pathology is recommended. Equivocal lesions should be managed in the same manner as atypical hyperplasia, i.e., continuous high-dose progestins (medroxyprogesterone acetate 20 to 40 mg by mouth daily) should be administered for 3 months. Endometrial biopsy is done at that time to demonstrate that the lesion is responding. If the lesion has been reversed within 6 months, ovulation induction can proceed. After the woman has completed her childbearing, hysterectomy should be performed.

Pelvic Relaxation

The woman with endometrial cancer who also requires surgery to correct symptomatic pelvic relaxation should have the corrective surgery done before radiation is administered. A combined vaginal and abdominal approach is employed unless repair work is needed only on the anterior vagina. In that instance, the abdominal approach alone is used. After the hysterectomy, the surgical bed and vagina are irrigated with saline or water before proceeding with the colporrhaphy. If radiation is given first, especially a course of external beam therapy with the usual 6-week waiting period, fibrosis with the resultant shrinkage can fix the vaginal and surrounding tissues, including the urethral-vesicle angle, preventing satisfactory repair.

Estrogen Replacement

Many women after treatment for endometrial cancer will suffer the effects of estrogen insufficiency, i.e., hot flushes, dyspareunia of vaginal dryness, and rapid loss of calcium from bone. Such women also are concerned about recurrent cancer and exhibit fear with respect to taking estrogens. Most will experience subjective improvement by taking medroxyprogesterone acetate 10 mg daily by mouth or 150 mg intramuscularly every 3 months. Should this prove ineffective, a low dose of conjugated estrogens, e.g., 0.3 or 0.625 mg daily, can be given in addition to the progestin. The progestin will prevent or minimize the possibility of a growth-enhancing estrogenic effect should there be any residual carcinoma. If the estrogen is not administered for 1 or 2 years after treatment, the risk of residual disease is very small.

REFERENCES

1. Boronow, R. C. (1973): Editorial comment—a fresh look at corpus cancer management. *Obstet. Gynecol.*, 42:448–451.
2. Boronow, R. C., Morrow, C. P., Creasman, W. T., DiSaia, P. J., and Blessing, J. A. (1982): Surgical-pathologic staging of FIGO Stage I endometrial carcinoma. *Obstet. Gynecol.*
3. Bean, H., Bryant, A., Carmichael, J. A., and Mallik, A. (1978): Carcinoma of the endometrium in Saskatchewan: 1966 to 1971. *Gynecol. Oncol.*, 6:503–514.
4. Creasman, W. T., DiSaia, P. J., Blessing, J., Wilkinson, R. H., Johnston, W., and Weed, J. C. (1981): Prognostic significance of peritoneal cytology in patients with endometrial cancer and preliminary data concerning therapy with intraperitoneal radio-pharmaceuticals. *Am. J. Obstet. Gynecol.*, 141:921–929.
5. Dahle, R. (1956): Transtubal spread of tumor cells in carcinoma of the body of the uterus. *Surg. Gynecol. Obstet.*, 102:332–336.
6. Heyman, J., Reuterwall, O., and Benner, S. (1941): The Radiumhemmet experience with radio-therapy in cancer of the corpus of the uterus. *Acta Radiol. (Diagn.) (Stock.)*, 22:14–98.
7. Kottmeier, H. L. (1968): Individualization of therapy in carcinoma of the corpus. In: *Cancer of the Uterus, Tubes and Ovaries, Proceedings of the 11th Annual Clinical Conference on Cancer, Houston, 1966*, pp. 102–108. Year Book Medical Publishers, Chicago.
8. Lewis, B. V., Stallworthy, J. A., and Cowdell, R. (1970): Adenocarcinoma of the body of the uterus. *J. Obstet. Gynaecol. Br. Commonw.*, 77:343–348.
9. Macasaet, M., Brigati, D., Boyce, J., Nicastri, A., Waxman, M., Nelson, J., and Fruchter, R. (1980): The significance of residual disease after radiotherapy in endometrial carcinoma: Clini-copathologic correlation. *Am. J. Obstet. Gynecol.*, 138:557–563.
10. Morrow, C. P., DiSaia, P. J., and Townsend, D. E. (1973): Current management of endometrial carcinoma. *Obstet. Gynecol.*, 42:399–405.
11. Morrow, C. P., and Schlaerth, J. B. (1982): Surgical management of endometrial carcinoma. *Clin. Obstet. Gynecol.*, 25:81–92.
12. Truskett, I. D., and Constable, W. C. (1968): Management of carcinoma of the corpus uteri. *Am. J. Obstet. Gynecol.*, 101:689–694.
13. Welander, C., Griem, M. L., Newton, M., and Marks, J. E. (1972): Staging and treatment of endometrial carcinoma. *J. Reprod. Med.*, 8:41–46.

Recent Clinical Developments in Gynecologic
Oncology, edited by C. Paul Morrow, et al.
Raven Press, New York © 1983.

Treatment of Advanced Endometrial Cancer with Tamoxifen and Aminoglutethimide

*M. A. Quinn, **J. J. Campbell, †R. Murray, and *R. J. Pepperell

*Department of Obstetrics and Gynaecology, University of Melbourne, Melbourne,
Australia; **Peter MacCallum Hospital, Melbourne, Australia; and †Endocrine Clinic,
Cancer Institute, University of Melbourne, Melbourne, Australia

The prognosis of patients with advanced endometrial carcinoma is poor, with 5-year survival rates of less than 40% for stage III tumours and 5 to 15% for stage IV tumours (9,21). Therapy for patients with advanced or recurrent disease at present is less than optimal and consists of local radiotherapy and the use of progestogens (3,19,26) or, more recently, cytotoxic agents (4,23).

Both endogenous and exogenous oestrogens have been implicated in the genesis of endometrial cancer. In patients with endometrial cancer, high circulating levels of oestrone and oestradiol (1,2) and increased urinary oestrogen excretion (25) have been reported, perhaps related to the increased conversion of androgens to oestrogens in such women as a result of obesity (5,15,18,24). With the knowledge that about 35% of cases of advanced endometrial carcinoma respond to progestogen therapy (3) and that such a tumour contains hormone receptors similar to those of breast carcinoma, as well as the enzymes necessary for physiological cyclical changes during the menstrual cycle (30), it is not unreasonable to consider endometrial tumours to be at least in part hormone dependent. A case can thus be made for using hormonal "manipulative" therapy similar to that currently used in patients with advanced breast carcinoma, such as tamoxifen therapy, adrenal ablation with surgery, or aminoglutethimide therapy.

Tamoxifen is a nonsteroidal antioestrogen, whose mode of action is as yet unclear (12); it may act by attaching to different areas of the receptor molecule from the oestradiol site and interfere with the binding of oestradiol, or it may modify the transfer of the oestradiol-receptor complex to the nucleus (16,17). It has been found to be a valuable agent in the treatment of patients with advanced breast cancer, with the notable absence of serious side effects (20,31). Binding of tamoxifen to oestrogen receptors in endometrial cancer has been demonstrated (14).

More than 30% of patients with advanced breast cancer respond to surgical adrenalectomy (8). Recent reports have confirmed the efficacy of aminoglutethimide in reducing adrenal steroid production by first blocking the conversion of cholesterol to pregnenolone and then inhibiting all adrenal steroid production (6). A selective inhibition of androstenedione aromatisation to oestrone is also evident (10), although appreciable circulating levels of oestrone are still detected during treatment (27). The use of this drug and appropriate replacement therapy in patients with disseminated breast cancer gives results comparable to adrenal surgery (22,28). A single case of advanced endometrial adenocarcinoma that has responded to surgical adrenalectomy has also been reported (13).

The aim of the study discussed in this chapter was to evaluate the efficacy of tamoxifen and aminoglutethimide alone or in combination in the treatment of patients with advanced endometrial carcinoma who had not responded to progestogen therapy or who had responded and then relapsed.

MATERIALS AND METHODS

Patients admitted to the study had stage III or IV endometrial cancer not responsive to medroxyprogesterone therapy; patients with local pelvic or abdominal recurrence were included only after appropriate megavoltage or surgical therapy had proven ineffective in controlling the disease. Eleven patients meeting these requirements were included in the study; informed consent was obtained in each case.

All patients were admitted to the hospital for preliminary assessment and initial therapy. Preliminary assessment included liver function tests, urea and electrolyte determinations, full blood examination, bone scan, liver scan, chest X-ray, and pelvic ultrasonography where applicable. Lymphangiography and computerised axial tomography were used in selected cases.

After being considered suitable for entry into the trial, patients were randomised with respect to treatment with either aminoglutethimide or tamoxifen. Aminoglutethimide was initially given in a dose of 250 mg twice daily, with a stepwise daily increase of 250 mg every 2 days until adrenal blockade was effected, as reflected in a reduction of plasma dehydroepiandrosterone sulphate to at least 50% of baseline value. Replacement therapy with cortisone acetate, 37.5 mg daily, was commenced simultaneously with aminoglutethimide. Fluorocortisone, 0.1 mg daily, was also prescribed, unless hypertension or peripheral oedema was present. Tamoxifen was given in a dose of 20 mg twice daily.

Patients were seen every 2 weeks as outpatients and evaluated after 8 weeks of treatment, when bone and liver scans, chest X-rays, and pelvic sonography were repeated. Where a complete or partial response was achieved, therapy was continued indefinitely and patients reviewed at monthly intervals. Where disease progressed, the alternate drug was added to the treatment regime, and patients were reviewed monthly. Assessment of response was as follows: (a) complete response: complete disappearance of all lesions during therapy; (b) partial response: a decrease of 50% or greater in the sum of the products of the two largest perpendicular diameters of all measurable lesions; (c) stable disease: a decrease of less than 50% in the sum of the products of the two largest perpendicular diameters of all measurable lesions; and (d) progressive disease: an increase in the size of measurable lesions.

RESULTS

Details of patients and response to therapy are shown in Table 1. Six patients were initially treated with tamoxifen; 1 patient (no. 9) had a complete response, 1 patient (no. 3) a partial response, and 4 patients had no response to treatment. Patient no. 3, who had a partial response and relapsed at 9 months, was changed to aminoglutethimide and again had a partial response. Of the 4 patients who failed to respond to tamoxifen, 2 had aminoglutethimide added to the treatment, 1 of whom (no. 5) is well after 14 months with stable disease and 1 of whom failed to respond; 1 patient was changed to aminoglutethimide alone, but the disease continued to progress; and 1 patient was so ill at the 8-week reevaluation that no further therapy was instituted.

Five patients were initially treated with aminoglutethimide. One patient (no. 8) had a complete response and 2 patients (nos. 2 and 11) had stable disease for 8 and 6 months, respectively. One of the 2 patients who failed to respond to aminoglutethimide had tamoxifen added to the treatment, but progression of the disease continued. Similarly, tamoxifen was added following a relapse in patient no. 2 but to no avail.

Toxicity

No patient experienced a drug rash, but lethargy was common in patients treated with aminoglutethimide. Two patients treated with aminoglutethimide experienced intermittent dizziness, and 1 of these fractured her femur in a fall during an episode of vertigo. Nausea caused by tamoxifen was sufficient enough to change treatment in 2 cases (nos. 1 and 3).

DISCUSSION

We have confirmed the antitumour activity of tamoxifen in patients with advanced endometrial cancer not responsive to medroxyprogesterone. Since commencement of this study, Swenerton et al. (29) have reported 4 responses in 7 patients treated with tamoxifen, all of whom had received medroxyprogesterone previously; 3 of the 4 responders had initially responded to medroxyprogresterone but subsequently relapsed, suggesting a different mechanism of tumour response to progestogens and tamoxifen. Of interest in our patients was the presence of oestrogen and progesterone receptors in the primary tumour of patient no. 9, who developed recurrent disease while on medroxyprogesterone and had a complete response to tamoxifen, and the absence of oestrogen and progesterone receptors in the secondary tumour of patient no. 3, who showed a partial response to both tamoxifen and aminoglutethimide. The absence of progesterone receptors in endometrial carcinoma has been shown to make a response to progesterone less likely but does not absolutely preclude it (7).

Our findings are the first results of the use of aminoglutethimide in patients with recurrent endometrial carcinoma, and they indicate that further study of this drug

TABLE 1. *Details of patients and response to treatment*

| Patient no. | Age | Initial findings | | | Time to recurrence | Site of recurrence | Treatment | Response | Comments |
		Stage	Histology	Invasion[a]					
1	61	Ib	G3	2/3	10 months	R. ischium, lungs	T	Progressed	Changed to AG→ progressed
2	74	II	G2	1/3	23 months	Liver, intra-abdominal	AG	Stable	Progressed at 8 months; T added→progressed
3	69	Ia	G1	2/3	7 months	Neck, mediastinum	T	Partial	Progressed at 9 months; changed to AG→ partial response
4	58	III	G3	2/3	7 years	Neck, pelvis	AG	Progressed	T added→ progressed
5	70	II	G2	?	5 years	R. pubic ramus, mediastinum	T	Progressed	AG added→ stable at 14 months
6	64	III	G2	3/3	2 years	Pelvis, paraaortic nodes	T	Progressed	AG added→ progressed
7	60	Ia	G3	3/3	1 year	Omentum, liver	T	Progressed	Died at 2 months
8	60	Ib	G1	1/3	14 months	Pelvis	AG	Complete	Well at 14 months
9	59	II	A/Sq	3/3	5 months	Pelvis	T	Complete	Progressed at 10 months
10	63	II	G2	?	3 years	Neck, mediastinum	AG	Progressed	Died at 5 months
11	59	Ib	G2	3/3	7 months	Paraaortic nodes	AG	Stable	Progressed at 6 months

[a]Invasion = depth of myometrial invasion by tumour. G1: well differentiated, G2: moderately well differentiated, G3: poorly differentiated, A/Sq: adenosquamous, T: tamoxifen, AG: aminoglutethimide.

in a clinical setting is warranted. It has been reported that the concentration of an antioestrogen must be 20 times that of oestrogen to exert its effect (11), so that by using aminoglutethimide to reduce circulating oestrogens concurrently with tamoxifen, a better therapeutic response may be achieved.

The relative lack of side effects of both drugs makes their use attractive in a population which is often elderly and less likely to tolerate cytotoxic chemotherapeutic agents.

ACKNOWLEDGMENTS

We are grateful to the Anti-Cancer Council of Victoria for a grant, to Ciba-Geigy for the aminoglutethimide and to Imperial Chemical Industries for the tamoxifen.

REFERENCES

1. Aleem, F. A., Moukhtar, M. A., Hung, W. C., and Romney, S. L. (1976): Plasma estrogen in patients with endometrial hyperplasia and carcinoma. *Cancer*, 38:2101–4.
2. Benjamin, F., and Deutsch, S. (1976): Plasma levels of fractionated estrogens and pituitary hormones in endometrial carcinoma. *Am. J. Obstet. Gynecol.*, 126:638–47.
3. Bonte, J. (1972): Medroxyprogesterone in the management of primary and recurrent or metastatic uterine adenocarcinoma. *Acta Obstet. Gynecol. Scand. Suppl.*, 19:21–4.
4. Bruckner, H. W., and Deppe, G. (1977): Combination chemotherapy of advanced endometrial adenocarcinoma with adriamycin, cyclophosphamide, 5-fluorouracil and medroxyprogesterone acetate. *Obstet. Gynecol. Suppl.*, 50:105–25.
5. Calanog, A., Sall, S., Gordon, G. G., and Southren, A. L. (1977): Androstenedione metabolism in patients with endometrial cancer. *Am. J. Obstet. Gynecol.*, 129:553–6.
6. Dexter, R. N., Fishman, L. M., Ney, R. L., and Liddle, G. W. (1967): Inhibition of adrenal corticosteroid synthesis by amino-glutethimide: Studies of the mechanism of action. *J. Clin. Endocrinol. Metab.*, 27:473–80.
7. Ehrlich, C. E., Young, P. C. M., and Cleary, R. E. (1977): Progesterone receptors—a new approach to recurrent endometrial cancer. *Proc. Am. Assoc. Cancer Res.*, 18:7–14.
8. Fracchia, A. A., Randall, H. T., and Farrow, J. H. (1967): The results of adrenalectomy in advanced breast cancer in 500 consecutive patients. *Surg. Gynecol. Obstet.*, 125:747–756.
9. Frick, H. C. II, Munnell, E. W., Richart, R. M., Berger, A. P., and Lawry, M. F. (1973): Carcinoma of the endometrium. *Am. J. Obstet. Gynecol.*, 115:663–672.
10. Gower, D. B. (1974): Modifiers of steroid-hormone metabolism: a review of their chemistry, biochemistry and clinical applications. *J. Steroid Biochem.*, 5(5):501–523.
11. Hahnel, R., Twaddle, E., and Ratajczak, T. (1973): The specificity of the estrogen receptor of human uterus. *J. Steroid Biochem.*, 4:21–31.
12. Hahnel, R., Twaddle, E., and Ratajczak, T. (1973): The influence of synthetic anti-estrogens on the binding of tritiated estradiol-17-beta by cytosols of human uterus and human breast carcinoma. *J. Steroid Biochem.*, 4:687–95.
13. Hubbard, T. B. Jr. (1960): The effect of adrenalectomy on adenocarcinoma of the uterus. *Cancer*, 13:1032–1034.
14. Jordan, V. C., and Koerner, S. (1975): Tamoxifen (ICI 46474) and the human carcinoma 8S oestrogen receptor. *Europ. J. Cancer*, 11:205–206.
15. Longcope, C., Pratt, J. H., Schneider, S. H., and Fineberg, S. E. (1978): Aromatization of androgens by muscle and adipose tissue in vivo. *J. Clin. Endocrinol. Metab.*, 46:146–152.
16. Lunan, C. B., and Green, B. (1973): Effect of compound ICI 46474 (Nolvadex) on the uptake of [^{3}H] oestradiol by human uterine endometrium. *Biochem. Soc. Transact.*, 1:500–502.
17. Lunan, C. B., and Green, B. (1974): ^{3}H-oestradiol uptake in vivo by human uterine endometrium: effect of tamoxifen (I.C.I. 46,474). *Clin. Endocrinol.*, 3:465–480.
18. MacDonald, P. C., Edman, C. D., Hemsell, D. L., Porter, J. C., and Siiteri, P. K. (1978): Effect of obesity on conversion of plasma androstenedione to estrone in postmenopausal women with and without endometrial cancer. *Am. J. Obstet. Gynecol.*, 130:448–455.

19. Malkasian, G. D. Jr., Decker, D. G., Jorgensen, E. O., and Webb, M. J. (1974): Evaluation of 6,17α-dimethyl-6-dehydroprogesterone for treatment of recurrent and metastatic gynecologic malignancy. *Am. J. Obstet. Gynecol.*, 118:461–465.
20. Manni, A., Trujillo, J. E., Marshall, J. S., Brodkey, J., and Pearson, O. H. (1979): Antihormone treatment of stage IV breast cancer. *Cancer*, 43:444–450.
21. Milton, P. J. D., and Metters, J. S. (1972): Endometrial carcinoma: an analysis of 355 cases treated at St. Thomas' Hospital (1945–69). *J. Obstet. Gynaecol. Br. Commonw.*, 79:455–464.
22. Newsome, H. H., Brown, P. W., Terz, J. J., and Lawrence, W. Jr. (1977): Medical and surgical adrenalectomy in patients with advanced breast carcinoma. *Cancer*, 39:542–546.
23. Piver, M. S., Lele, S., and Barlow, J. J. (1980): Melphalan, 5-Fluoro-uracil, and medroxyprogesterone acetate in metastatic or recurrent endometrial carcinoma. *Obstet. Gynecol.*, 56:370–372.
24. Rizkallah, T. H., Tovell, H. M. M., and Kelly, W. G. (1975): Production of estrone and fractional conversion of circulating androstenedione to estrone in women with endometrial carcinoma. *J. Clin. Endocrinol. Metab.*, 40:1045–1056.
25. Rome, M., Brown, J. B., Mason, T., Smith, M. A., Laverty, C., and Fortune, D. (1977): Oestrogen excretion and ovarian pathology in postmenopausal women with atypical hyperplasia, adenocarcinoma and mixed adenosquamous carcinoma of the endometrium. *Br. J. Obstet. Gynaecol.*, 84:88–97.
26. Rozier, J. C. Jr., and Underwood, P. B. Jr. (1974): Use of progestational agents in endometrial adenocarcinoma. *Obstet. Gynecol.*, 44:60–64.
27. Samojlik, E., Santen, R. J., and Wells, S. A. (1977): Adrenal suppression with aminoglutethimide. II. Differential effects of aminoglutethimide in plasma androstenedione and estrogen levels. *J. Clin. Endocrinol. Metab.*, 45:480–487.
28. Santen, R. J., Samojlik, E., Lipton, A., Harvey, H., Ruby, E. B., Wells, S. A., and Kendall, J. (1977): Kinetic, hormonal and clinical studies with aminoglutethimide in breast cancer. *Cancer*, 39:2948–2958.
29. Swenerton, K. D., Shaw, D., White, G. W., and Boyes, D. A. (1979): Treatment of advanced endometrial carcinoma with tamoxifen. *N. Engl. J. Med.*, 301:105.
30. Tseng, L., Gusberg, S. G., and Gurpide, E. (1977): Estradiol receptors and 17 beta-dehydrogenase in normal and abnormal human endometrium. *Ann. N.Y. Acad. Sci.*, 286:190–198.
31. Ward, H. W. C. (1973): Anti-oestrogen therapy for breast cancer: a trial of tamoxifen at two dose levels. *Br. Med. J.*, 1:13–14.

Recent Clinical Developments in Gynecologic Oncology, edited by C. Paul Morrow, et al. Raven Press, New York © 1983.

Basis for Hormonal Manipulation of Gynecologic Tumors

William E. Gibbons[1] and Timothy J. O'Brien

Department of Obstetrics and Gynecology, University of Southern California School of Medicine, Los Angeles, California 90033

The understanding of the mechanism of steroid hormone action has resulted in a logical and successful hormonal approach to the treatment of breast carcinoma. The application of these concepts to the management of gynecologic neoplasia is a more recent development, but the body of information in this area is continuously growing. A review of the proposed mechanism of action of steroid hormones will aid in our understanding of recent advances in endocrinologic therapy of pelvic neoplasia.

Steroid hormones circulate in the blood both bound to serum proteins and unbound, or "free." It is the free hormone that is available for simple diffusion across cell membranes, although the role of hormone-specific serum-binding proteins is being reevaluated. Steroid-sensitive target tissues (Fig. 1) contain intracytoplasmic binding proteins (receptors), which are specific for each steroid. The hormone binds to its receptor, enabling the hormone-receptor complex to translocate into the nucleus and bind to chromatin. This initiates the synthesis of mRNA (transcription). Messenger RNA serves as the protein code for new protein synthesis, which occurs in the alteration of cell function, that is, the steroid effect (5). For example, one of the proteins whose synthesis is stimulated by estrogen is the estrogen receptor itself. Thus, estrogen can increase the cell sensitivity for its own subsequent stimulation.

Steroid hormones also modulate the effect of other steroid hormones. Progesterone antagonizes estrogen action by blocking the synthesis of estrogen receptor. It does this by utilizing its own specific cytoplasmic receptor system. Figure 2 demonstrates levels of progesterone- and estrogen-receptor molecules present in the uterus under the influence of various hormones. These levels can be increased by the administration of estrogens and reduced to near basal levels by the coadministration of progesterone. Figure 2 also demonstrates that androgens, which also

---

[1]*Present address*: Department of Obstetrics and Gynecology, Baylor University School of Medicine, Houston, Texas 77027.

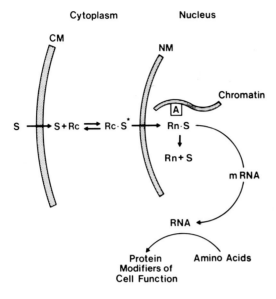

FIG. 1. Proposed mechanism of hormone action. S: steroid hormone; Rc: cytoplasmic receptor; S*: activated receptor; CM: cell membrane; NM: nuclear membrane; Rn: nuclear translocated receptor; A: acceptor site; mRNA: messenger ribonucleic acid.

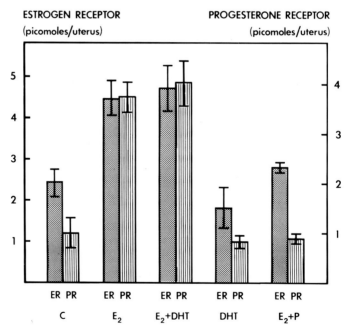

FIG. 2. Effect of progesterone and dihydrotestosterone on estrogen-stimulated increases in estrogen- and progesterone-receptor concentrations. ER:estrogen receptor; PR:progesterone receptor; C: control; E_2: estradiol treatment group; E_2 + DHT: estradiol + dihydrotestosterone treatment group; DHT: dihydrotestosterone treatment group; E_2 + P: estradiol + progesterone treatment group.

antagonize estrogen action, do not appear to mediate this effect by reducing the levels of estrogen or progesterone receptors.

The value of measuring receptor levels in hormone-responsive tissues is evident upon the review of breast-cancer data. The initial question asked of breast lesions by researchers is whether or not they contain estrogen receptor. About two-thirds of breast carcinomas contain measurable levels of estrogen receptor, and similar concentrations are found in the metastatic lesions, as well as in the primary lesions (12). This is important if treatment directed at disseminated disease is to be based on the measurement of primary-lesion receptor levels. It was subsequently observed that the presence of estrogen receptors could be used to predict whether or not a tumor will respond to hormonal manipulation. Paone et al. (15) observed (Table 1) that 70% of estrogen-receptor-positive tissues responded to hormonal therapy, compared to 14% that had undetectable levels (5). The reasons why 30% of receptor-positive tumors do not respond and why some receptor-negative tumors do are many. The presence of receptors in the cytoplasm does not mean that they will translocate and bind in the nucleus, that once in the nucleus they can initiate transciption, or that all normally responsive genes will be responsive in a less-differentiated tumor.

There is also a positive correlation of hormonal-therapy response with the presence of estrogen receptor in the nuclear compartment (11). Furthermore, if progesterone receptor, which is a product of estrogen stimulation, could be measured, it would suggest a functional estrogen-receptor system. Brooks et al. (3) reported a 66% response rate in tumors that are both estrogen- and progesterone-receptor-positive versus 28% of tumors with estrogen receptor only. The data must be interpreted in light of the estrogen milieu. Without estrogen stimulation there would be no nuclear accumulation and no stimulation of estrogen- or progesterone-receptor levels. This can explain why some apparently estrogen-receptor-negative tissues respond to subsequent hormonal therapy.

STERIOD HORMONE RECEPTORS IN GYNECOLOGIC NEOPLASMS

Receptor levels have been measured in gynecologic neoplasms. Our studies on endometrial carcinomas (Table 2) indicate that many such tumors contain both estrogen and progesterone receptors. It also appears that more differentiated lesions

TABLE 1. *Relationship between breast-cancer receptor status and response to hormonal therapy*

Breast-carcinoma estrogen-receptor status	Patients with positive response	
	%	No. positive response/total no.
Positive	70	23/33
Negative	14	3/22

From Paone et al. (15), with permission.

TABLE 2. *Estrogen- and progesterone-receptor levels in normal and carcinomatous endometrium*

Tissue	Grade	No.	Cytosol estrogen-receptor level		Cytosol progesterone-receptor level	
			% positive	fmol/mg protein[a]	% positive	fmol/mg protein[a]
Adenocarcinoma	I	4	75	120	100	670
Adenocarcinoma	II	16	62	64	68	161
Adenocarcinoma	III	15	27	37	33	80
Benign proliferative endometrium		12	85	63	92	364
Adenomatous hyperplasia		3	100	335	67	675

[a]Average value.

have a greater proportion of receptor-positive tissues and a higher concentration of receptor per tumor than less differentiated lesions. Crocker et al. (6), Grilli et al. (9), Muechler et al. (14), Pollow et al. (16), and others have also noted both progesterone and receptor levels in a high percentage of endometrial carcinomas. Ehrlich et al. (8), as well as Crocker, noted higher receptor positivity in more differentiated lesions. Mortel et al. (13) reported a positive correlation between serum estradiol and measurable levels of progesterone receptor, which points to normal nuclear handling of estrogen receptor in many of the tumors. Mortel observed the following: had not nuclear receptor been evaluated in his series, 13% of the lesions would have been considered receptor negative.

Ovarian neoplasms may also contain hormone receptor. Holt et al. (10) observed the presence of estrogen receptor or progesterone receptor in 8 of 16 tumors (mucinous and serous cystadenocarcinomas). He was unable to correlate histologic grade with receptor level. Our results from a small number of tumors demonstrate (Table 3) that measurable levels of estrogen and/or progesterone receptor were frequently observed. There was a tendency for the endometrioid lesions to show a higher percentage of receptor-positive tumors than the serous or mucinous form. Receptor levels from cervical carcinomas also suggest that the more differentiated the lesion, the greater the likelihood of measuring estrogen and/or progesterone receptor in the cytoplasm of the tumor (Table 4).

TABLE 3. *Estrogen- and progesterone-receptor levels in ovarian carcinoma*

Histologic type	No.	Cytosol estrogen-receptor level		Cytosol progesterone-receptor level	
		% positive	fmol/mg protein[a]	% positive	fmol/mg protein[a]
Serous	4	0	0	0	0
Mucinous	3	33	25	0	0
Endometrioid	4	50	57	0	0
Undifferentiated	4	25	9	50	30

[a]Average value.

TABLE 4. *Estrogen- and progesterone-receptor levels in cervical cancer*

Tumor	No.	Cytosol estrogen-receptor level		Cytosol progesterone-receptor level	
		% positive	fmol/mg protein[a]	% positive	fmol/mg protein[a]
Squamous, differentiated	19	26	19	26	87
Squamous, poorly differentiated	11	9	3	27	13
Adenocarcinoma	4	25	12	100	123

[a]Average value.

Progestins have long been used to treat advanced metastatic endometrial adenocarcinomas with varying degrees of success. The correlation of receptor status with hormonal response reported for breast lesions has not been as completely established with endometrial lesions. Since more-differentiated endometrial adenocarcinomas appear more likely to respond to progestin therapy and to have receptor present, a direct relationship is suggested. Ehrlich et al. (8), in reviewing their results of receptor assay and its relationship to progestin therapy, found that 7 of 8 progesterone-receptor-positive tumors responded to progestin therapy, while only 1 of 15 tumors without measurable progesterone receptor demonstrated a response, i.e., reduction in tumor size. Their report summarizes the results of a series where tumor response and receptor status is compared. Ninety-four percent of progesterone-positive tumors (30 of 32) responded to progestin therapy, whereas only 11% of tumors (4 of 38) without progestin receptor responded to progestins. Most importantly, the receptor status was a better predictor of progestin response than the degree of differentiation.

A new form of hormonal therapy recently applied to gynecologic neoplasia involves a class of agents known as antiestrogens. Antiestrogens are defined as nonsteroidal compounds that antagonize estrogen properties and stimulate gonadotropin output from the pituitary gland. They are capable of binding to cytoplasmic estrogen receptor and translocating the receptor to the nucleus, where they are retained for prolonged periods. As a result, there is reduced synthesis of new estrogen receptor, which decreases the ability of the tissue to respond normally to estrogen exposure. Tamoxifen, an antiestrogen, opposes estrogen-promoted growth, as does progesterone. Moreover, the administration of tamoxifen can measurably increase progesterone-receptor levels. When tamoxifen has been used in the treatment of breast cancer in premenopausal patients with estrogen-receptor-positive (ER+) tumors, response rates are in the range of 50% (1,11). In addition, results correlate with the presence of cytoplasmic levels of estrogen receptor, indicating that tamoxifen is utilizing a normal estrogen mechanism of action. The cytotoxic effect of tamoxifen was studied in uterine adenocarcinomas in tissue culture by Sekiya and Takamizawa (20). Both tamoxifen and clomiphene resulted in reduced colony formation. The addition of progesterone brought about a synergistic effect in further reducing colony formation. This occurs because progesterone and tamoxifen use different receptors and because tamoxifen, like estrogens, stimulates the synthesis of progesterone receptor. When Mortel and co-workers evaluated the effects of tamoxifen on human adenocarcinoma receptor levels, he observed that with the oral administration of tamoxifen, estrogen-receptor levels were not significantly affected, whereas there was a significant increase in progesterone receptor in 73% of tumors. In 4 tumors, which were initially progesterone-receptor-negative, tamoxifen therapy induced significant progesterone-receptor concentrations.

There have been a few published studies where antiestrogen therapy was utilized in endometrial carcinoma. Bonte et al. (2) evaluated short-term tamoxifen therapy *in vitro* and *in vivo*. They found that 50 mg of tamoxifen taken by mouth daily for 7 days resulted in a transformation of the endometrial glands from a pseudostratified appearance to a monolayered, atrophic glandular structure. This also occurred in tissue culture. Medroxyprogesterone acetate (MPA) therapy resulted in reduced cytoplasmic estrogen-receptor concentrations as expected. MPA reduced cytoplasmic progesterone binding, whereas tamoxifen therapy increased progestin binding levels. Bonte et al. treated 17 postmenopausal endometrial cancer patients with 40 mg tamoxifen a day. All had previously received progestin therapy. Results were evaluated after the patients had been treated for at least 3 months. Complete response was defined as the complete disappearance of the tumor, and partial response was defined as the decrease of the bulk tumor size by 50% and no development of new disease during the course of therapy. The duration of the response had to be at least 2 months. Of the 17 patients, a complete regression occurred in 2 and a partial regression in 7. However, the duration of response was only 3 months, compared to the 15 months observed in patients treated with progestin. A relationship was suggested between the response to progestin and the response to tamoxifen. If the patients had responded previously to progestin, there was greater likelihood of a positive tamoxifen response (Table 5).

Swenerton (21) evaluated tamoxifen therapy in 10 patients with endometrial carcinoma. Using criteria similar to those noted above, he observed a complete response in 1 patient, a partial response in 2, stable disease in another 2, and progression in 5. A response to tamoxifen also correlated with (a) a previous response to progestins and (b) a "disease-free interval" between initial therapy and a recurrence interval of greater than 2 years. More differentiated lesions had a higher response rate than lesions with less differentiation. Eighty-six percent of the grade II lesions responded to tamoxifen, compared to 25% of the grade III lesions. Furthermore, in 3 patients who had "escaped" tamoxifen response and who had

TABLE 5. *Relationship of progestin response to tamoxifen response in therapy of endometrial adenocarcinoma*

Response to progestin	No.	Response to tamoxifen			
		Complete	Partial	Stabilization	Progression
Complete	4	1	3	0	0
Stabilization	4	0	3	0	1
Unsuccessful	4	0	1	0	3

From Bonte et al. (2), with permission.

previously responded and "escaped" progestin therapy, a response was induced by combination progestin-tamoxifen therapy. This suggests that a recovery of the progestin response was induced by the tamoxifen therapy, possibly through the promotion of progesterone-receptor synthesis.

Side effects of tamoxifen therapy are generally uncommon and mild. They include nausea, vomiting, skin rash, hot flashes, vaginal bleeding, hypercalcemia (rare), and myelosuppresion (rare). The reported number of patients with breast or endometrial carcinomas who have to discontinue therapy is small. The role of tamoxifen therapy in the treatment of endometrial carcinoma appears assured for a variety of reasons. Tamoxifen utilizes a different site of action than progestins in inhibiting neoplastic growth; it also appears to induce tissue progesterone-receptor levels, which may increase the sensitivity of the tumor to progestin therapy and may also serve as a predictor of tumor response, and it has low toxicity. However, the short duration of response observed in some studies suggests that tamoxifen's main role may be in combination with progestins.

In summary, pelvic neoplasms, not unexpectedly, contain steroid receptors. The concentration of receptors in edometrial carcinoma correlates with the degree of differentiation. Progestin-therapy response correlates with the presence of progesterone receptor and, more importantly, appears to correlate with progesterone-receptor presence better than with the degree of differentiation. This underscores the need for receptor studies in endometrial carcinoma, since the information will help direct therapy, as in breast cancer. Tamoxifen, an antiestrogen, may have a significant future as adjuvant hormonal therapy combined with progestins in the treatment of endometrial carcinoma.

MÜLLERIAN-INHIBITING SUBSTANCE

A promising new form of hormonal therapy for müllerian neoplasia utilizes müllerian-inhibiting substance (MIS). The MIS is secreted by fetal testes and has been shown to cause regression of the ipsilateral müllerian (paramesonephric) duct system in males. Morphologic and ultrastructural studies demonstrate that its initial onset of action is manifested as an alteration of the duct epithelium and surrounding mesenchyma (17), thus suggesting both endocrine and paraendocrine effects. Extracts containing MIS activity obtained by bioassay techniques result in ovarian cortical atrophy when incubated with embryonic ovarian tissue (18). Since the majority of neoplasms are of epithelial origin and arise from cortical elements, the possibility of therapeutic application exists. Donahoe et al. (7), who have been working with MIS for a decade, have observed cytotoxicity within human ovarian cancer cell lines by incubating them with extracts of fetal calf testes. This exposure to MIS resulted in the cell death of actively growing cells in the S_1 stage of the cell cycle, where there is active replication of DNA. In addition, testicular extracts incubated in tissue culture of human endometrial carcinomas demonstrated dose-related cytotoxicity (19). At present, even with such advanced techniques as affinity chromatography, a pure form of MIS has not been isolated and characterized (4). A monoclonal antibody to bovine MIS has recently been reported (22). While future therapy of gynecologic cancer with MIS is anticipated, thus far there have been no human clinical trials.

REFERENCES

1. Bloom, N. D., Tobin, E. H., Schreibman, B., and Degenshein, G. A. (1980): The role of progesterone receptors in the management of advanced breast cancer. *Cancer*, 45:2992.
2. Bonte, J., Ide, P., Billiet, G., and Wynants, P. (1981): Tamoxifen as a possible chemotherapeutic agent in endometrial adenocarcinoma. *Gynecol. Oncol.*, 11:140.
3. Brooks, S. C., Saunders, D. E., Singhakowinta, A., and Vaitkevicius, V. K. (1980): Relation of tumor content of estrogen and progesterone receptors with response of patient to endocrine therapy. *Cancer*, 46:2775.
4. Budzik, G. P., Swann, D. A., Hayashi, A., and Donahoe, P. K. (1980): Enhanced purification of müllerian inhibiting substance by lectin affinity chromatography. *Cell*, 21:909.
5. Chan, L., and O'Malley, B. W. (1978): Steroid hormone action: Recent advances. *Ann. Intern. Med.*, 89:694.
6. Crocker, S. G., Milton, P. J., and King, R. J. (1974): Uptake of 6,7³H-estradiol, 17β by normal and abnormal human endometrium. *J. Endocrinol.*, 62:145.
7. Donahoe, P. K., Swann, D. A., Hayashi, A., and Sullivan, M. D. (1979): Müllerian duct regression in the embryo correlated with cytotoxic activity against human ovarian cancer. *Science*, 205:913.
8. Ehrlich, C. E., Young, P. C. M., and Cleary, R. E. (1981): Cytoplasmic progesterone and estradiol receptors in normal, hyperplastic, and carcinomatous endometria: Therapeutic implications. *Am. J. Obstet. Gynecol.*, 141:539.
9. Grilli, S., Ferrari, A. M., Gola, G., Rochetta, R., Orlandi, C., and Prodi, G. (1977): Cytoplasmic receptors for 17β-estradiol, 5α-dihydrotestosterone and progesterone in normal and abnormal human uterine tissue. *Cancer Lett.*, 2:247.
10. Holt, J. A., Caputo, T. A., Kelly, K. M., Greenwald, P., and Chorost, S. (1979): Estrogen and progestin binding in cytosols of ovarian adenocarcinomas. *Obstet. Gynecol.*, 53:50.
11. Leake, R. E., Laing, L., Calman, K. C., Macbeth, F. R., Crawford, D., and Smith, D. C. (1981): Oestrogen-receptor status and endocrine therapy of breast cancer: Response rates and status stability. *Br. J. Cancer*, 43:59.
12. Leclercq, G., Henson, J. C., Doboel, M. C. Legros, N., Longeual, E., and Mattheiem, W. H. (1977): Estrogen and progesterone receptors in human breast cancer. In: *Progesterone Receptors in Normal and Neoplastic Tissues*, edited by W. L. McGuire, p. 141. Raven Press, New York.
13. Mortel, R., Levy, C., Wolff, J. P., Nicolas, J. D., Robel, P., and Baulier, E. E. (1981): Female sex steroid receptors in postmenopausal endometrial carcinoma and biochemical response to an antiestrogen. *Cancer Res.*, 41:1140.
14. Muechler, E. K., Flinckinger, G. L., Mangan, C. E., and Mikhail, G. (1975): Estradiol binding by human endometrial tissue. *Gynecol. Oncol.*, 3:244.
15. Paone, J. F., Abeloff, M. D., Ettinger, S. S., Arnold, E. A., and Baker, R. R. (1981): The correlation of estrogen and progesterone receptor levels with response to chemotherapy for advanced carcinoma of the breast. *Surg. Gynecol. Obstet.*, 152:70.
16. Pollow, K., Boquoi, E., Lubbert, H., and Pollow, B. (1975): Effect of gestagen therapy upon 17β hydroxysteroid dehydrogenase in human endometrial carcinoma. *J. Endocrinol.*, 67:131.
17. Price, J. M., Donahoe, P. K., and Ito, Y. (1979): Involution of the female müllerian duct of the fetal rat in the organ-culture assay for the detection of müllerian inhibiting substance. *Am. J. Anat.*, 156:265.
18. Rashedi, M., Stoll, R., and Maraud, R. (1976): Inhibiting effect of the testis on the ovary of the chick embryo. *C. R. Soc. Biol.*, 170:756.
19. Rosenwaks, Z., Liu, H. C., Jones, H. W., Tseng, L., and Stone, M. L. (1981): *In vitro* inhibition of endometrial cancer growth by a neonatal rat testicular secretory product. *J. Clin. Endocrinol. Metab.*, 52:817.
20. Sekiya, S., and Takamizawa, H. (1976): The combined effect of nonsterodial anti-oestrogens and sex steroids on the growth of rat uterine adenocarcinoma cells in tissue culture. *Br. J. Obstet. Gynaecol.*, 83:183.
21. Swenerton, K. D. (1980): Treatment of advanced endometrial adenocarcinoma with tamoxifen. *Cancer Treat. Rep.*, 64:805.
22. Vigier, B., Picard, J. Y., and Josso, N. (1982): A monoclonal antibody against bovine antimüllerian hormone. *Endocrinol.*, 110:131.

Recent Clinical Developments in Gynecologic
Oncology, edited by C. Paul Morrow, et al.
Raven Press, New York © 1983.

Steroid Receptor Analysis and the Clinical Management of Breast Cancer

*K. Griffiths, *R. I. Nicholson, *B. Joyce, *M. Morton,
**C. Campbell, and **R. W. Blamey

*Tenovus Institute for Cancer Research, Cardiff, CF4 4XN Wales; and **The City
Hospital, Nottingham, NG5 1PB England

It has long been established that the growth and functional activity of various tissues concerned with the female reproductive processes are dependent on the synthesis and secretion of oestrogens by the ovary. It was recognised that atrophy of vaginal epithelium and the uterus occurred after castration, and many years ago Beatson (3) indicated that the growth rate of carcinoma of the female breast could be controlled by oophorectomy. Only intensive research over the past two decades has allowed us to begin to understand the biochemical mechanisms by which oestrogens and other steroid hormones regulate the biological processes of these hormone-dependent tissues. It is now well accepted that in the breast cell, as in other steroid-responsive target tissues (18,29), the hormone functions through a well-defined series of intracellular events, initiated by the association of oestradiol-17β with its cytoplasmic receptor protein and followed by the translocation of the steroid-receptor complex to the nucleus. There it is bound to specific nuclear acceptor sites in chromatin and promotes the various transcriptional events resulting in the synthesis of macromolecular components, such as mRNA and rRNA, that are essential for cell maintenance and function. This concept of hormone dependence, essentially a process that maintains an effective intracellular concentration of oestradiol-receptor (ER) complex at a site at which it may influence gene expression, is based on early pioneering experiments of Jensen and co-workers (21,22,24), which established the mechanism by which such tissues are able to concentrate steroids.

METASTATIC BREAST CANCER

It must now be recognised that this particular programme of research into the mechanism of steroid action has been responsible for certain advances in our approach to the management of patients with breast cancer. Since the early work of Beatson, endocrine therapy, either ablative or additive, has been considered the effective form of treatment for advanced metastatic cancer of the breast, although it is also accepted that the objective response rate in general has only been of the order of 30%. However, it was very apparent that the ER content of breast tumour tissue may provide a predictive test for the selection of patients with advanced disease for endocrine therapy, and the early analyses of De Sombre et al. (15) and Jensen et al. (23) clearly suggested that such a concept would be substantiated.

Indeed, the results from many centres throughout the world (28,32,33) have provided unequivocal evidence that the steroid-receptor content of metastatic tissue offers a valuable guide to the clinician concerned with the management of patients with advanced breast cancer. The majority of patients (94%) whose tissue did not contain ER, failed to respond to endocrine therapy, whereas approximately 50% of those with ER-positive tumour tissue responded well to such treatment. Of those who had failed to respond but were ER positive, it would seem that the receptor may be present in the cytoplasm of the tumour but translocation may not occur, or possibly the binding of the ER complex to acceptor sites is defective. However, evidence is also available indicating that the response can be even more reliably predicted when the amount of the oestrogen receptor present in the tissue is considered (33); the higher the ER concentration the greater the response rate.

Thus, the data clearly indicate that patients with advanced breast cancer with ER-negative tumour tissue rarely respond to endocrine therapy. Evidence is also accumulating suggesting that analysis of the tumour tissue for both oestrogen receptor and progesterone receptor (PR) may improve the predictive capacity of such tests and more effectively identify patients who respond to this form of therapy (13,28). The concept that certain tissues require "oestrogen priming" before progesterone can produce any biological response has long been accepted in reproductive physiology. The investigations of Horwitz and co-workers (26) indicated that the synthesis of PR was dependent on oestrogen acting through the ER system. It therefore seems that the presence of receptor for progesterone in breast cancer reflects the functional integrity of the complete oestrogen-response mechanism. Approximately 80% of women with advanced stages of the disease whose tumour tissue contained receptors for oestradiol and progesterone responded to endocrine therapy (31).

To date, evidence relating to the association between ER status of metastatic tissue and response to chemotherapy remains equivocal (13). Although Lipmann and co-workers (30) suggested that patients with ER-positive tumours respond less favourably to chemotherapy, Kiang et al. (27) failed to confirm this, and more results are needed before the prognostic value of receptor analyses can be assessed in relation to chemotherapy.

STEROID RECEPTOR STATUS OF PRIMARY BREAST CANCER

Receptor analysis has proven to be of value in the treatment of advanced disease, but despite the reported success of such work, it is clear that not all metastatic deposits are readily available for biopsy. In many instances, only primary tumour tissue obtained at mastectomy would be available for receptor analysis. It therefore was necessary to evaluate the relationship between the ER status of primary breast tumours and the natural history of the disease and to assess its prognostic value in relation to the disease-free interval, the response to endocrine therapy upon recurrence, the site of metastatic spread, and ultimate survival (Fig. 1). The following

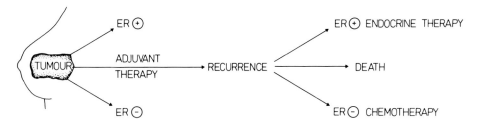

FIG. 1. Schematic representation of natural history of carcinoma of breast.

discussion deals with such a study, instituted in 1973 by the Breast Clinic of The City Hospital in Nottingham, England, and the Tenovus Institute for Cancer Research in Cardiff, Wales.

Patients and Receptor Analyses

A total of 550 patients, all without evidence of distant metastases and with tumours less than 5 cm in diameter, presented consecutively to one surgeon (R. W. B.) between 1973 and 1979. Treatment involved a simple or subcutaneous mastectomy, and biopsies were taken of lymph nodes in the lower axilla and the apex of the axilla and from the internal mammary chain. Patients without histologically evident tumour in any node were classified stage A, those with tumour in the lower axilla only as stage B, and those in whom the apex of the axilla or internal mammary chain was involved as stage C. Tumours were graded by Dr. C. Elston of The City Hospital according to Bloom and Richardson (8); grade 1 was the most differentiated, and grade III, the least. Patient follow-up was carried out at regular intervals, and no patient received any systemic adjuvant therapy, treatment being withheld until the disease had recurred.

Tumour tissue was immediately frozen after removal and stored in liquid nitrogen until transported in dry ice to Cardiff for analysis of the oestrogen-receptor status as previously described (36).

ER Status and Natural History of Disease

It is now well established that approximately 60% of breast tumours contain measurable amounts of oestrogen receptor (32). It is also accepted that the ER status reflects the degree of tumour differentiation, the histological grade of the tumour correlating well with receptor content (13,16,35) and the majority of undifferentiated grade III tumours being ER negative. No correlation has yet been established between ER status and tumour size and between ER status and the disease stage (13).

Data from the Nottingham study clearly confirm earlier reports (8,12,41) that tumour grade (Fig. 2c), as well as stage (Fig. 2a) and tumour size (Fig. 2b), can be a useful guide to eventual disease recurrence. Of interest was the relationship between ER status and recurrence. Earlier results (34) showed that tumours in patients with ER-negative primary breast tumours tended to recur quickly; furthermore, when survival was considered (4), an advantage was also observed for women

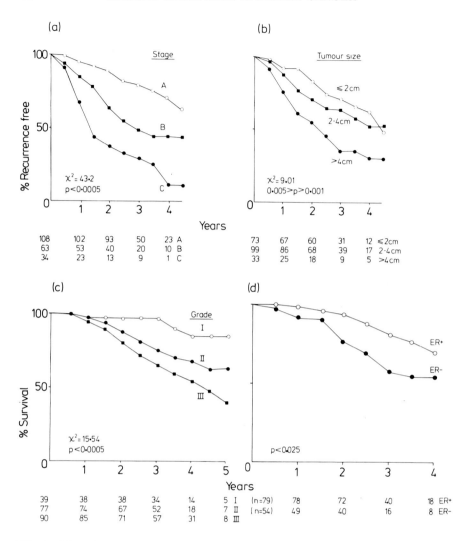

FIG. 2. Life table analysis curves established from data derived each succeeding time. Differences between curves are compared (Haybittle and Freedman, ref. 20). Relationship shown between lymph-node status and tumour size with recurrence-free interval and between tumour grade and ER status with survival.

with tumours containing measurable levels of receptor (Fig. 2d). However, the practical value of ER status alone as a prognostic parameter must be limited, since the correlations are not sufficiently strong for the reasonably accurate prediction of recurrence for any individual patient, and ultimately the association between ER status and other clinical parameters in a prognostic index would appear to offer a more effective approach (6).

This has been supported by the accumulating and recently reported (36) data from the Nottingham study. Patients with no tumour involvement of the nodes (stage A) formed a "good prognosis" group (6), with 85% overall survival after 4 years regardless of the receptor status. On the other hand, early recurrence was evident (Fig. 3) in patients with nodal involvement and ER-negative tumours, especially when the higher nodes (stage C) were involved. Approximately 70% of the stage C patients with ER-negative tumours died within 3 years. Although patients with axillary node involvement (stages B and C combined) and ER-positive tumours generally fared better than those with ER-negative tumours, with nearly 70% surviving 3 years (Fig. 4), it was interesting that in this group of patients, it was the women with grade III tumours who formed the "bad prognosis" group (Fig. 5). The survival rate of this group was similar to all patients with nodal involvement and ER-negative tumours (Fig. 6a). Patients with ER-positive tumours and nodal involvement with grade I or II tumours did as well as all stage A patients (Fig. 6b). It might well be asked therefore whether ER status and grade are both required as prognostic indicators. Histological grade is, however, a subjective assessment about which few pathologists express confidence. The receptor analysis is an objective measurement, especially when it is the responsibility of a specialised, experienced laboratory excercising effective quality control procedures and must be recommended as an integral part of the laboratory information available to the clinician managing patients with breast carcinoma. The Nottingham study and similar investigations conducted throughout the world provide good evidence that

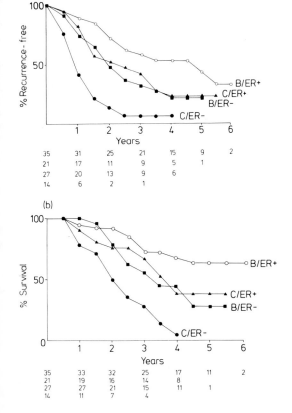

FIG. 3. ER status and disease-free interval and survival in lymph-node-positive patients.

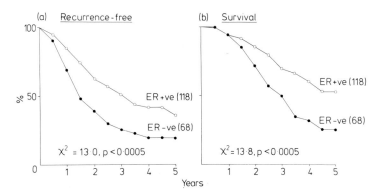

FIG. 4. Relationship between oestrogen-receptor status and prognosis in patients with nodal involvement (stages B and C).

ER analysis, together with other clinical parameters, can predict the natural history of the disease and offers a rational basis for patient selection for adjuvant therapy.

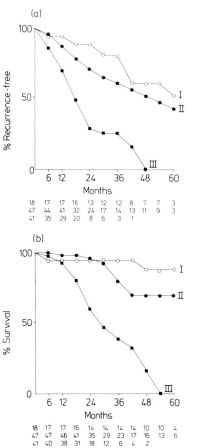

FIG. 5. Relationship between tumour grade and prognosis in patients with nodal involvement and ER-positive tumours.

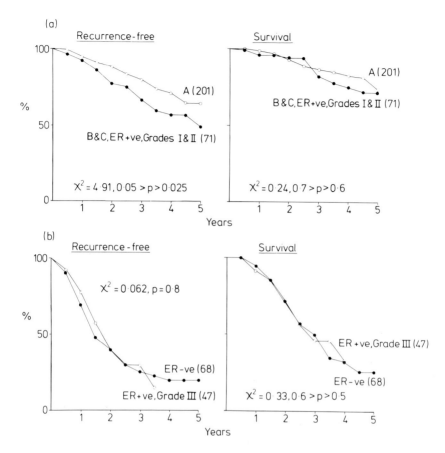

FIG. 6. **(a)** Relationship between patients without nodal involvement (stage A) and those with nodal involvement (stages B and C) and grade I and grade II tumours. **(b)** Prognosis of patients with nodal involvement. Comparison of patients with ER-negative tumours and those with ER-positive grade III tumours.

ER Status: Site of Recurrence and Response to Therapy

In the Nottingham study, local recurrence of the disease is defined as multiple symptomatic or progressive metastases in mastectomy flaps requiring major treatment. Regional recurrence is considered symptomatic metastases in axillary or supraclavicular nodes requiring therapy (36). The anatomical site of distant metastasis has been considered a valuable prognostic factor relating to therapy response (2) and to survival (14,39). Patients with skeletal metastases respond better to endocrine therapy than those with secondary spread to the viscera. Although ER status did not relate to local recurrence, the incidence of symptomatic regional recurrence was greater in patients with poorly differentiated grade III tumours or ER-negative tumours (Table 1). Moreover, the site of distant metastasis was also found to relate to both ER status and tumour grade, with ER-positive tumours tending to spread to bone and with the ER-negative, undifferentiated cancer metastasising to the viscera (Table 2).

TABLE 1. *ER status, histological grade, and major regional recurrence*

	ER status[a]			Histological grade[b]			
	Positive	Negative	Total	I	II	III	Total
Recurrence	20	29	49	2	9	38	49
No recurrence	244	166	410	77	187	202	466
Total	264	195	459	79	196	240	515

[a]$\chi^2 = 6.3$; 1 df; $p < 0.05$.
[b]$\chi^2 = 21.1$; 2 df; $p < 0.001$.

Furthermore, evidence is now becoming available indicating that the ER status of the primary tumour will predict the patient response to endocrine therapy should the disease recur (7,13). The Nottingham results support this. Of the 55 patients with ER-positive primary tumours treated with endocrine therapy, oophorectomy (if premenopausal), or tamoxifen (if postmenopausal), 17 patients (31%) responded, whereas 2 of 40 (5%) of the ER-negative patients were shown by external assessment to have an objective response. Equally interesting and in accord with earlier studies of McGuire and co-workers (33) on the analysis of metastatic breast cancer, the response rate appears to increase with increasing concentration of receptor in the cytosol of the primary tumour (Fig. 7).

NEW RECEPTOR ASSAYS

Patient selection for various treatment schedules would seem possible from the knowledge of the ER status of the primary tumour. There is little recorded evidence of marked changes in receptor phenotype in the period between mastectomy and disease recurrence (13,28). Therefore, the high-risk patients can be identified for appropriate adjuvant therapy after mastectomy, and the ER status of the primary tumour is valuable in treating the recurring disease.

Essential to this concept, of course, is that the receptor assay is reliable and effectively quality controlled (40), and it is the considered opinion of many experts in the field (9) that experienced regional laboratories should be responsible for such

TABLE 2. *ER status, site, and total incidence of distant metastases*

	ER status			Histological grade			
	Positive	Negative	p	I	II	III	p
Site of first distant recurrence							
Bone	42	13	<0.001	7	21	26	ns
Viscera	17	36	<0.001	2	10	42	<0.001
Combined	10	6	ns	1	7	8	ns
Total	69	55	ns	10	38	76	<0.01
No recurrence	195	140		69	158	164	

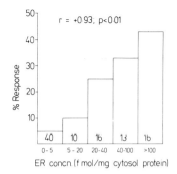

FIG. 7. Relationship between response to endocrine therapy of patients with recurrent disease and ER status of primary tumour. Data indicate number of patients with variable amounts of estrogen receptor in primary tumour; histogram indicates percentage of patients responding to treatment.

analysis. Certainly, a technician in a basic, clinical chemistry laboratory would generally find it extremely difficult to maintain good quality analysis when handling small batch numbers of receptor assays at irregular intervals.

The principles of receptor analysis have been described in detail numerous times (10) and the various procedures considered in detail (32). It is now generally accepted (13) that the multiple-point, dextran-coated charcoal (DCC) assay for oestrogen receptor is the more reliable procedure, providing reasonable precision. Details of the assay used in the studies reported in this chapter have been described (36). The quality of the assay can be maintained only if strict attention to methodological detail is adhered to and if adequate internal quality control is practised. Unless the assay is undertaken immediately, tumour tissue should be rapidly frozen after surgical removal. The preparation and handling of tissue cytosol is important. Internal quality control is probably best achieved using aliquots of lyophilised tissue, such as calf uterus or human myometrium, and an obvious control factor that can be imposed on the analytical system is the value of the dissocation constant K_D. This is clearly a fundamental thermodynamic property of the basic chemical reaction between oestradiol and receptor, and, as such, the value should be constant, changing only under the influence of irregularities associated with each stage of the analysis. When such effects cause the K_D to fall outside preset arbitrary limits, the analytical results are unacceptable.

Another important aspect of quality control concerns the protein concentration of the cytosol, a parameter against which receptor levels are generally related. Errors associated with protein estimation can often be far greater than realised and, as such, can markedly distort the basic errors of receptor-site determination when expressed as units/mg cytosol protein.

This type of assay is expensive and relatively time consuming, and there are now reports in the literature (13) on the use of comparatively simple histochemical procedures involving the binding of oestrogen-fluorescein conjugates to tissue sections. Potentially such procedures offer certain advantages, primarily the identification of the cells in a heterogeneous breast tumour that do or do not contain receptor. A wide spectrum of such conjugates have been assessed, including oestradiol-fluorescein amine; oestradiol linked at various C positions and through different bridging groups to fluorescein; and oestradiol linked to bovine serum albumin fluorescein isothiocyanate (BSA-FITC). Despite reports indicating the effectiveness of such procedures in localising oestrogen receptors (13) and the correlation of histochemistry with conventional receptor assays, the ability of the technique to identify the receptor has been the subject of some controversy, and Chamness and co-workers (11) were unable to support the contention that such fluorescein conjugates visualise oestrogen receptor.

Our own research (25) over the past 3 years supports the concern expressed by these authors. Special emphasis in the investigation was given to the purity of various oestrogen-fluorescein conjugates, the relative binding affinities (RBA) of which were assessed by competition between conjugate and ^{3}H-oestradiol-17β in a standard rat uterine cytosol preparation. The ability of the conjugate to bind the cytosol receptor and displace ^{3}H-oestradiol was determined over a wide range of concentrations. The conjugates tested displayed some degree of competition for sites on the receptor (Table 3), although the binding affinity was low compared to oestradiol-17β or diethylstilboestrol. This was especially true of fluorescein conjugates linked to oestradiol-17β via BSA, or where horseradish peroxidase had been attached to the steroid molecule. Pretreatment of the BSA conjugate with DCC immediately prior to its use in competition studies decreased the apparent affinity of the receptor for the conjugates by more than tenfold. The purity of the conjugate is clearly important in such studies, since contaminating-free oestradiol would displace the tritiated label and suggest binding of the conjugate to receptor. However, it is interesting that the same intensity of fluorescence was seen when the oestradiol-BSA-FITC conjugates were used, both pre- and post-DCC stripping, for the histochemical visualisation of receptor (25). The introduction of a hexamethylenediamine bridging group at the C-17 position of oestradiol-17β to increase the

TABLE 3. *Relative binding affinities of various steroid-fluorescein conjugates in rat uterine cytosol assay*

Competitor	Relative binding affinity %	
Oestradiol-17β	100	
Diethylstilboestrol	94	
Oestrone-17-FA	2.8	
Oestradiol-17-FA	1.4	
Ethynyloestradiol-6-FA	0.6	
Oestradiol-17-HMD-FA	0.6	
Oestradiol-6-FA	0.2	
Oestradiol-17-HRP	0.04	
Testosterone-17-FA	<0.01	
5α-Dihydrotestosterone-17-FA	<0.01	
Progesterone-11α-FA	<0.001	
	Charcoal treatment	
	−	+
Oestradiol-6-BSA-FITC	0.01	<0.001
Oestradiol-17-BSA-FITC	0.01	<0.001
Progesterone-11α-BSA-FITC	<0.001	<0.0001

FA: fluorescein amine, HMD: hexamethylenediamine (bridge), BSA: bovine serum albumin, FITC: fluorescein isothiocyanate, HRP: horseradish peroxidase.

distance between fluorescein and the steroid molecule reduced the affinity for the receptor. Conjugates with direct links to the oestradiol molecule gave the highest relative binding affinity.

Histochemical results obtained after treatement *in vivo* of oestrogen target tissues with either oestradiol or tamoxifen have been compared with the cellular location of oestrogen-receptor protein determined using ^{3}H-oestradiol exchange assays previously described (38). Two types of tissue from Sprague Dawley rats were used: (a) uteri from 1-week ovariectomised animals were removed two hr after intravenous administration of saline vehicle, oestradiol-17β (5 μg), or tamoxifen (300 μg) and (b) dimethylbenzanthracene(DMBA)-induced mammary tumours from intact animals, which were treated as in (a). After sacrifice, some tissue samples were taken for histochemical localisation procedures, and the remainder, for total and accessible oestrogen-receptor site concentrations (37,38) in cytosol and nuclear fractions.

Uteri from ovariectomised rats contained high levels of cytoplasmic oestrogen receptor (813 fmole/uterus, $N = 5$) and low nuclear concentration (203 fmole/uterus, $N = 5$) when assayed by standard procedures on homogenised preparations. Histochemical procedures, using oestradiol-17β-fluorescein amine conjugate, gave a similar pattern with predominantly cytoplasmic fluorescence (Fig. 8). Fluorescence in sections of DMBA-induced mammary tumour was also primarily localised in epithelial cytoplasm.

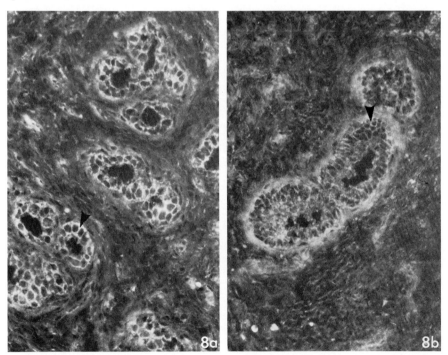

FIG. 8. Histochemical localisation of oestrogen-binding proteins in sections (4 mμ) of rat uterus incubated with oestradiol-17-fluorescein amine (×125). Arrow indicates distinct rim of fluorescence in cytoplasm of glandular epithelial cells.

It is interesting that a similar fluorescent pattern was obtained by incubation with fluorescein-labelled progesterone or 5α-dihydrotestosterone.

Injection of animals with oestradiol or tamoxifen 2 hr prior to sacrifice resulted in a shift of receptor from the cytoplasm (233 fmole/uterus and 329 fmol/uterus, respectively) to the nucleus (774 fmole/uterus and 532 fmol/uterus, respectively) as determined biochemically. Histochemically, only conjugates linked through BSA, i.e., those with the lowest RBA, produced nuclear fluorescence patterns (Fig. 9) both pre- and post-DCC stripping. The remainder of the conjugates studied continued to demonstrate cytoplasmic binding fluorescence. A fourfold increase in the concentration of the conjugate in the histochemical medium failed to produce nuclear fluorescence.

It was also disappointing that when a series of human breast-tumour samples were studied, once again only cytoplasmic fluorescence was observed with all conjugates and no clear correlation was found between the ER status of the tumour, measured biochemically, and the fluorescent staining. Evidence from these and other studies undertaken over the past few years at the Tenovus Institute indicates that the histochemical procedures currently used do not identify the receptor protein normally measured by saturation analysis. Perhaps the histochemical procedures

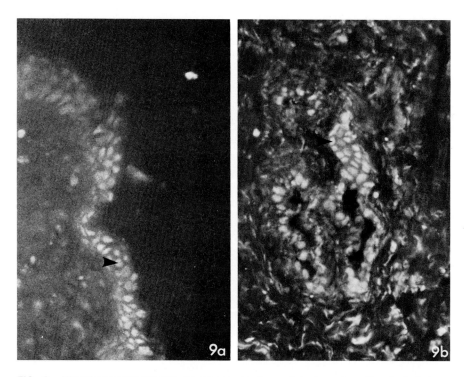

FIG. 9. Histochemical localisation of oestrogen-binding proteins in sections (4 mμ) of rat uterus incubated with oestradiol-6-(O-carboxymethyl)-oxime-BSA-FITC conjugate (×125). Arrow indicates nuclear fluorescence in lumen **(a)** and glandular **(b)** epithelial cells, respectively.

effectively localise a second class of oestrogen-binding protein, as described by Eriksson et al. (17).

This may eventually be seen to relate to hormone dependence, but work is required to correlate the results to the clinical situation. As stressed by Chamness and co-workers (11), extensive efforts by the histochemist must be made to validate the technique before it can even be suggested that the procedures may replace the conventional biochemical analyses of receptor content.

More appropriate may be a radiometric assay for the receptor protein, which has been in reasonably pure form by at least two laboratories (1,19). The work in Dr. Jensen's laboratory is well advanced, with excellent antiserum raised against the receptor protein, and reports indicate that a procedure for its measurement by radiometric assay may soon be available. This would determine total receptor concentration but will also have to be validated for clinical purposes against conventional assays. Furthermore, an immunocytochemical procedure to localise receptor protein by using this antiserum and a horseradish peroxidase label will clearly offer a technique with considerable potential for research into the biochemistry of breast cancer.

ACKNOWLEDGMENT

The authors are grateful to the Tenovus Organisation for generous financial support.

REFERENCES

1. Al-Nuaimi, N., Davies, P., and Griffiths, K. (1979): Purification of the cytoplasmic oestrogen receptor from mammary tumours induced in rats with dimethylbenzanthracene. *J. Endocrinol.*, 81:119–130.
2. Baum, M. (1980): The management of advanced breast cancer. *Br. J. Hosp. Med.*, 23:32–38.
3. Beatson, G. T. (1896): *Lancet*, 2:104 and 162.
4. Bishop, H. M., Blamey, R. W., Elston, C. W., Haybittle, J. L., Nicholson, R. I., and Griffiths, K. (1979): Relationship of oestrogen receptor status to survival in breast cancer. *Lancet*, 2:283–284.
5. Blamey, R. W., Bishop, H. M., Blake, J. R. S., Doyle, P. J., Elston, C. W., Haybittle, J. L., Nicholson, R. I., and Griffiths, K. (1980): Relationship between primary breast tumour receptor status and patients survival. *Cancer*, 46:2765–2769.
6. Blamey, R. W., Elston, C. W., Haybittle, J. L., Nicholson, R. I., and Griffiths, K. (1983): Prognostic factors in the Nottingham-Tenovus breast cancer study. In: *Commentaries in Breast Cancer*, edited by J. Taylor and R. Bulbrook. 3:*(in press)*.
7. Block, G. E., Ellis, R. S., de Sombre, E. R., and Jensen, E. V. (1978): Correlation of estrophilin content of primary mammary cancer to eventual endocrine treatment. *Ann. Surg.*, 188:372–376.
8. Bloom, H. J. G., and Richardson, W. W. (1957): Histological grading and prognosis in breast cancer. *Br. J. Cancer*, 11:359–369.
9. British Breast Group (1980): Steroid-receptor assays in human breast cancer. *Lancet*, 1:298–300.
10. Chamness, G. C. and McGuire, W. L. (1979): Methods for analysing steroid receptors in breast cancer. In: *Breast Cancer, Vol. 3*, edited by W. L. McGuire, pp. 149–197. Plenum Press, New York.
11. Chamness, G. C., Mercer, W. D., and McGuire, W. L. (1980): Are histochemical methods for estrogen receptor valid? *J. Histochem. Cytochem.*, 28:792–798.
12. Champion, H. R., Wallace, I. W., and Prestcott, R. I. (1972): Histology in breast cancer prognosis. *Br. J. Cancer*, 26:129–136.
13. Consensus Meeting on Steroid Receptors in Breast Cancer, N.I.H., Washington (1980): *Cancer*, 46: no. 12.
14. Cutler, S. J., Asim, A. J., and Taylor, S. G. (1969): Classification of patients with disseminated cancer of the breast. *Cancer*, 24:861–869.

15. De Sombre, E. R., Smith, S., Block, G. E., Ferguson, D. J., and Jensen, E. V. (1974): Prediction of breast cancer response to endocrine therapy. *Cancer Chemother. Rep.*, 58:513–519.

16. Elston, C. W., Blamey, R. W., Johnson, J., Bishop, H. M., Haybittle, J. L., and Griffiths, K. (1980): The relationship of oestradiol receptor and histological tumour differentiation with prognosis in human primary breast carcinoma. In: *Breast Cancer, Experimental and Clinical Aspects*, edited by H. T. Mourisden and T. Palshof, pp. 59–62. Pergamon Press, Oxford and New York.

17. Eriksson, H., Upchurch, S., Hardin, J. W., Peck, E. J., and Clark, J. H. (1978): Heterogeneity of estrogen receptors in the cytosol and nuclear fractions of the rat uterus. *Biochem. Biophys. Res. Commun.*, 81:1–7.

18. Griffiths, K., Davies, P., Harper, M. E., Peeling, W. B., and Pierrepoint, C. G. (1979): The etiology and endocrinology of prostatic cancer. In: *Endocrinology of Cancer, Vol. II*, edited by D. P. Rose, pp. 1–56. CRC Press, Boca Raton, Florida.

19. Green, G. L., Nolan, C., Engler, J. P., and Jensen, E. V. (1980): Monoclonal antibodies to human estrogen receptor. *Proc. Natl. Acad. Sci. U.S.A.*, 77:5115–5119.

20. Haybittle, J. L., and Freedman, L. S. (1979): *Statistician*, 28:199.

21. Jensen, E. V., and de Sombre, E. R. (1973): Estrogen-receptor interaction. *Science*, 182:126–134.

22. Jensen, E. V., Jacobson, H. I., Flesher, J. W., Soha, N. N., Gupta, G. N. Smith, S., Colucci, V., Shiplacoff, D., Neumann, H. G., de Sombre, E. R. and Jungblut, P. W. (1966): Estrogen receptors in target tissues. In: *Steroid Dynamics*, edited by G. Pincus, T. Nakao, and J. F. Tait, pp. 133–147. Academic Press, New York.

23. Jensen, E. V., Polley, T. Z., Smith, S., Block, G. E., Ferguson, D. J., and de Sombre, E. R. (1975): Prediction of hormone dependency in human breast cancer. In: *Estrogen Receptors in Human Breast Cancer*, edited by W. L. McGuire, P. P. Carbone, and E. P. Vollmer, pp. 37–56. Raven Press, New York.

24. Jensen, E. V., Suzuki, T., Kawashima, T., Stumpf, W. E., Jungblut, P. W., and de Sombre, E. R. (1968): A two-step mechanism for the interaction of estradiol with rat uterus. *Proc. Natl. Acad. Sci. U.S.A.*, 59:632–638.

25. Joyce, B. G., Nicholson, R. I., Morton, M., and Griffiths, K. (1982): Studies with steroid-fluorescein conjugates on oestrogen-target tissues. *Eur. J. Cancer*, 18:1147–1155.

26. Horwitz, K. B., McGuire, W. L., Pearson, O. H., and Segaloff, A. (1975): Predicting response to endocrine therapy in human breast cancer: A hypothesis. *Science*, 189:726–727.

27. Kiang, D., Frenning, T., Goldman, D. R., Ascensao, V., and Kennedy, V. J. (1978): Estrogen receptors and response to chemotherapy and hormone therapy in advanced breast cancer. *N. Engl. J. Med.*, 299:1330–1334.

28. King, R. J. B. (editor) (1979): *Steroid Receptor Assays in Human Breast Tumours*. Alpha Omega Publishing, Cardiff.

29. King, R. J. B., and Mainwaring, W. I. P. (editors) (1974): *Steroid Cell Interactions*. Butterworths, London.

30. Lipmann, M. E., Allegra, J. C., Thompson, E. B., Simon, R., Barlock, A., Green, L., Huff, K. K., Do, H. M. T., Aitken, S., and Warren, R. (1978): The relation between estrogen receptors and response rate to cytotoxic chemotherapy in metastatic breast cancer. *N. Engl. J. Med.*, 298:1223–1228.

31. McGuire, W. L. (1980): Steroid hormone receptors in breast cancer treatment strategy. *Recent Prog. Horm. Res.*, 36:135–156.

32. McGuire, W. L., Carbone, P. P., and Vollmer, E. P. (editors) (1975): *Estrogen Receptors in Human Breast Cancer*. Raven Press, New York.

33. McGuire, W. L., Zata, D., Horwitz, K. B., and Chamness, G. C. (1978): Hormones, receptors and breast cancer. In: *Tumour Markers, Proceedings of the 6th Tenovus Workshop*, edited by K. Griffiths, A. M. Neville, and C. G. Pierrepoint. Alpha Oemega Publishing, Cardiff.

34. Maynard, R. V., Blamey, R. W., Elston, C. W., Haybittle, J. L., and Griffiths, K. (1978): Oestrogen receptor assay in primary breast cancer and early recurrence of the disease. *Cancer Res.*, 38:4292–4295.

35. Maynard, P. V., Davies, C. J., Blamey, R. W., Elston, C. W., Johnson, J., and Griffiths, K. (1978): Relationship between oestrogen receptor content and histological grade in human primary breast tumours. *Br. J. Cancer*, 38:745–748.

36. Nicholson, R. I., Campbell, F. C., Blamey, R. W., Elston, C. W., George, D., and Griffiths, K. (1981): Steroid receptors in early breast cancer: value in prognosis. *J. Steroid Biochem. (in press)*.

37. Nicholson, R. I., Davies, P., and Griffiths, K. (1977): Effects of oestradiol-17β and tamoxifen on nuclear oestradiol-17β receptors in DMBA-induced rat mammary tumours. *Eur. J. Cancer*, 13:201–208.
38. Nicholson, R. I., Golder, M. P., Davies, P., and Griffiths, K. (1976): Effects of oestradiol-17β and tamoxifen on total and accessible cytoplasmic oestradiol-17β receptors in DMBA-induced rat mammary tumours. *Eur. J. Cancer*, 12:711–717.
39. Papaioannou, A. N., Tany, F. J., and Volk, H. (1967): Fate of patients with recurrent carcinoma of the breast. *Cancer*, 20:371–376.
40. Wilson, D. W., Nix, A. R. J., Rowlands, R. J., Kemp, K. W., and Griffiths, K. (1981): Accuracy, precision and monitoring of error in quality control schemes. In: *Quality Control in Clinical Endocrinology*, edited by D. W. Wilson, S. J. Gaskell, and K. W. Kemp. Alpha Omega Publishing, Cardiff *(in press)*.
41. Wolff, B. (1966): Histological grading in carcinoma of the breast. *Br. J. Cancer*, 20:36–40.

Recent Clinical Developments in Gynecologic
Oncology, edited by C. Paul Morrow, et al.
Raven Press, New York © 1983.

Adjuvant Chemotherapy in Sarcoma of the Uterus: A Preliminary Report

Per Kolstad

Department of Gynaecology, The Norwegian Radium Hospital, Oslo 3, Norway

Sarcomas of the uterus are rare. In Norway there are approximately 10 cases a year, which constitutes an incidence of 0.5/100,000, which is comparable to the rates found in other parts of the Western world. Almost all cases detected in Norway are referred to the Norwegian Radium Hospital, either for primary treatment or for secondary treatment after surgery had been performed elsewhere. Since uterine sarcomas are so rare, the experience gained even in a large cancer-referral institution is still quite limited.

Since 1968, we have conducted two clinical studies on the value of irradiation and chemotherapy, and the results of the two studies are discussed below.

CLASSIFICATION

Histological diagnosis of uterine sarcomas can be difficult to make, and earlier reports have been rather confusing, since different histologists have used different criteria for determining malignancy. The most commonly used classification for uterine sarcomas today is that first proposed by Ober in 1959 (2) and later modified by Kempson (1). Ober suggested that uterine sarcomas be categorized according to their cell type and site of origin. Tumors can be either pure or mixed, the latter being composed of more than one cell type. Homologous tumors contain tissue elements entirely indigenous to the uterus, whereas heterologous tumors contain tissue elements that are foreign to the uterus. Because many of the sarcomas included in Ober's classification are extremely rare, we have followed the Gynecologic Oncology Group in the United States by simplifying the classification as shown in Table 1. The leiomyosarcomas in the table, as well as the endometrial stromal sarcomas and the mixed homologous müllerian sarcomas, all contain tissue found in the normal uterus, while the mixed heterologous müllerian sarcomas, also called mixed mesodermal tumors, contain tissue that is alien to the uterus.

Rhabdomyosarcoma (sarcoma botryoides) is the most common pure heterologous sarcoma. A rare tumor, it can occur at all ages but is primarily seen in young girls. In the two studies presented here, there is no such tumor. The incidence of malignant

TABLE 1. *Classification of uterine sarcomas*

Leiomyosarcomas
Endometrial stromal sarcomas
Mixed homologous müllerian sarcomas
(carcinosarcoma)
Mixed heterologous müllerian sarcomas
(mixed mesodermal sarcoma)
Other uterine sarcomas

mixed müllerian tumors is thought to be increasing, and at our hospital such tumors are encountered as often as leiomyosarcomas. The origin of mixed müllerian tumors has still not been clarified. One theory claims that such tumors arise from embryonal rests, while another theory, which is more commonly accepted, claims that such tumors are derived from the mesenchymal cells lying just below the endometrial epithelium. These tumors contain both carcinomatous and sarcomatous elements. Some believe that the homologous tumors, i.e., those containing only one sarcomatous element normally found in the uterus, have a better prognosis. It is impossible in these cases to predict which tissue will metastasize, but it is again thought that the sarcoma element is more malignant.

All the sarcomas found in the uterus may spread by contiguous growth, hematological spread, or lymphogenous spread. The most commonly used histopathological criteria for the determination of malignancy are hypercellularity, nuclear atypism, and/or prominent mitotic activity. At our hospital, we followed the recommendation that the number of mitoses per 10 high-power field (hpf) should be counted. Our experience has also shown that this is a reasonable means of separating tumors with very definite malignant potential from those that are more benign. The borderline is 5 mitoses per 10 hpf. Anything below this value means that the prognosis is good, and consequently the tumor may be considered benign. When more than 20 mitoses per 10 hpf are found, all patients eventually die, as has been corroborated by several series.

MATERIAL AND METHODS

At the Norwegian Radium Hospital, the sarcoma material has been reassessed twice in previous years but the results never published. The first series lasted from 1947 to 1962, when treatment was based on surgery, either alone or combined with external irradiation to the pelvic field. During most of these years, conventional radiotherapy with a four-field technique was used. High-voltage machines were introduced in 1957–58, and since then we have used either betatron or irradiation with cobalt machines or linear accelerators. A 5-year survival rate for the group in which the surgical borders were not free of malignancy or the sarcoma had already spread to other organs was only 7%. In the second study, which lasted from 1968 to 1974, actinomycin D was added as a radiosensitizer; It was also felt that this drug possibly could kill some tumor cells circulating in the body. At the time the second study was begun, actinomycin D was considered one of the possible drugs to be used in adjuvant therapy of sarcomas.

Table 2 shows the data from the 1947–62 and 1968–74 series. As can be seen from the table, actinomycin D did not produce better results. The sequence of therapy is shown in Table 3. When metastases were found during surgery or if radical surgery was impossible, several combined treatment schemes were used with little success.

The age distribution in a more recent series, from 1976 to 1980, shows that today women with sarcoma are slightly younger than women in previous years. Among the leiomyosarcoma patients, 7 were premenopausal; the average age of this group, which comprised 20 cases, was 51 years. The average age of women with endometrial stromal sarcoma was 53, and 5 were premenopausal, while the average age of those with mixed mesodermal tumors was 59, and 3 were premenopausal. The most common presenting symptoms are shown in Table 4. In the series from 1968 to 1974 the vast majority initially consulted a physician because of bleeding alone or bleeding with discharge. We found, as has been stressed by many authors, that the diagnosis in most patients with mixed mesodermal tumors can be established as a result of curettage, which was not the case in patients with leiomyosarcomas, in which case the operative specimen was often needed to make the final diagnosis.

As already mentioned, the results with combined actinomycin D and irradiation therapy had little effect on the survival rate. The most important factor that influenced survival was whether or not the tumor was localized in the uterus at the time of surgery. From Table 5 we can see that more than 50% of patients with a localized tumor survived for more than 5 years. In patients with nonlocalized tumors, only 2 of 33 cases are still alive today.

We have also sought to establish if mixed müllerian sarcomas are more malignant than leiomyosarcomas. Figure 1 shows the 5-year survival curve (calculated by the

TABLE 2. *Data on 1947–1962 and 1968–1974 series*

	1947–1962		1968–1974	
Type of sarcoma	Total no. cases	No. alive	Total no. cases	No. alive
Leiomyosarcoma	58	14	39	6
Endometrial stromal sarcoma	0	0	7	6
Mixed müllerian sarcoma	33	11	26	4
Unclassified	9	0	1	0
Total	100	25	73	16

TABLE 3. *Therapy sequence in localized disease for 1968–1974 series*

Radical surgery
Actinomycin D, 0.5 mg i.v. q.d. × 4 d.
Irradiation, 2,000 rads, pelvic field
Actinomycin D, 0.5 mg i.v. q.d. × 4 d.
Irradiation, 2,000 rads, pelvic field

TABLE 4. *Symptoms of uterine sarcomas*

Symptom	%
Bleeding and/or discharge	96
Pain	1
Increasing girth	1
Urinary symptoms	1
Routine examination	1

TABLE 5. *Uterine sarcomas, 1968–1974 series[a]*

Type of tumor	Total no. patients	No. alive
Localized tumor	40	21
Nonlocalized tumor	33	2
Total	73	23

[a]Treatment: surgery, radiation, actinomycin D.

actuarial method), from which we can see that the prognosis is as poor for leiomyosarcomas as for mixed müllerian sarcomas. Only approximately 30% survived for 5 years. Figure 1 also shows both localized and nonlocalized tumors. For localized tumors with operative borders free of involvement, the 5-year survival rate was about 50%.

It was sad to see that combined treatment did not produce any better results than in the earlier series. We began searching for other drugs; in the meantime, adriamycin had become available in our country. In 1975 we decided that all patients with localized sarcomas should receive adjuvant chemotherapy. We prescribed 60 mg/m^2 adriamycin, administered through a running intravenous flow every third

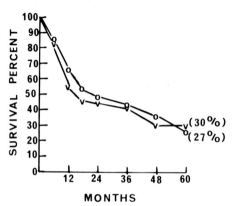

FIG. 1. Survival curves for mixed müllerian sarcoma and leiomyosarcoma (1968–74 series) treated with surgery, irradiation, and actinomycin D. o = Mixed müllerian sarcoma; v = leiomyosarcoma.

week, and the maximum dose to be received by any patient was approximately 500 mg/m². This required the patients' presence in a hospital every third week for approximately 7 to 9 months, when the maximum dose was reached.

We feel somewhat uneasy about presenting our data at this time, but the differences in the results between patients receiving actinomycin D and irradiation and patients receiving adriamycin is so marked that we would like more groups to institute such treatment. Omura and Blessing (3) have already shown that adriamycin alone can provide a 27% response rate in recurrent disease. We know of several trials currently under way in Scandinavia and other European countries, as well as in the United States, both with adriamycin alone or in combination with dimethyltriazenoimidazole carboxamide (DTIC) or other drugs. Figure 2 shows a comparison between the series receiving adriamycin and the series of localized tumors treated in the period from 1968 to 1974. We have closely monitored all patients. The longest follow-up period is now more than 4 years. In the group treated with adriamycin, which comprised 29 patients, only 3 died from their cancer: 1 of the 3 refused treatment, 1 died shortly after the start of treatment from lung metastases, and 1 died within 8 months from the time adjuvant chemotherapy was instituted. After 18 months, there was no recurrence in this group. In the group receiving actinomycin D and irradiation, which comprised 42 patients, 11 died from local recurrence, 8 from lung metastases, and 4 from other distant metastases.

In Fig. 3 we have divided the patients in the 1968–74 series into different histopathological groups. We can see from the figure that leiomyosarcomas seem to have the best prognosis, while mixed müllerian tumors have the poorest, with a 70% survival rate after 18 months. We have established 18 months as the limit for when new recurrences can appear, since we have observed that after this time lapse few die from their disease. In other words, if patients are recurrence-free after

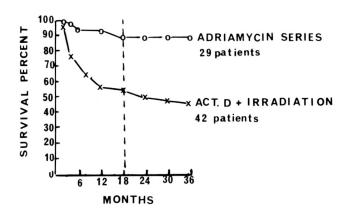

FIG. 2. Survival curves for patients receiving adjuvant treatment with adriamycin compared with patients receiving irradiation and actinomycin D.

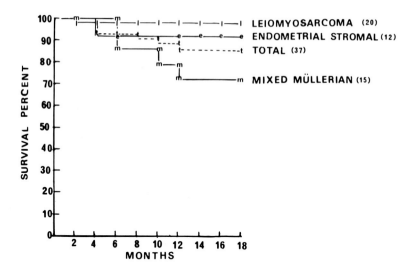

FIG. 3. Survival curves for patients with different types of uterine sarcomas (1976–80 series), all of whom received adjuvant treatment with adriamycin.

18 months, the prognosis should be very good. The 18-month survival for the adriamycin series is about 85%, which is far better than in the 1947–62 and 1968–74 series.

DISCUSSION

We would like to emphasize once again that the findings presented here are preliminary. There are some histopathological factors that must be reviewed again. In the series with adjuvant adriamycin treatment, it seems that endometrial stromal tumors occurred more frequently than in the earlier series. Furthermore, we want to examine atypia and, especially, the mitotic rate to ascertain if they are of any importance in adjuvant treatment. We will, of course, continue our series with adriamycin treatment in sarcomas of the uterus. We were asked by a Swedish group of gynecologic oncologists to join in a randomized trial, but having compared the above data with data in the literature and in our earlier series, we thought it unethical to stop giving our patients adriamycin. Nevertheless, we are extremely interested in learning of any other groups that wish to present their results in uterine sarcoma at this time.

In this chapter we have only dealt with localized tumors and adjuvant chemotherapy in such cases. We are also conducting studies on advanced disease using a combination of cyclophosphamide, actinomycin D, adriamycin, and vincristine. Thus far we have observed the disappearance of leiomyosarcomas in a number of patients receiving such combined treatment; 2 of these patients remain alive more than 3 years after treatment was stopped.

REFERENCES

1. Kempson, R. L., and Bari, W. (1970): Uterine sarcomas: Classification, diagnosis and prognosis. *Hum. Pathol.*, 1:331–342.
2. Ober, W. B. (1959): Uterine sarcomas: Histogenesis and taxonomy. *Ann. N. Y. Acad. Sci.*, 75:568–574.
3. Omura, G. A., and Blessing, J. A. (1978): Chemotherapy of stage III, IV and recurrent uterine sarcomas; a randomized trial of Adriamycin versus Adriamycin + DTIC. *AACR Abstract No. 103, Proceedings of AACR/ASCO.*

*Recent Clinical Developments in Gynecologic
Oncology*, edited by C. Paul Morrow, et al.
Raven Press, New York © 1983.

Müllerian Mixed Tumours of the Uterus

Patrick Finian Lynch

Coombe Lying-in Hospital, Dublin, Ireland

Some malignant tumours of the endometrium and other parts of the lower genital tract in women contain a mixture of epithelial and mesenchymal tissues, with or without elements foreign to the location in which they are found. Such tumours have been referred to by a confusing variety of names, including mixed mesodermal tumour (or mesodermal mixed tumours), carcinosarcoma, sarcoma botryoides, carcinosarcomatoides, and mesenchymal sarcoma. The use of the term "müllerian mixed tumour" has been recommended by the World Health Organisation (4). Müllerian mixed tumours are subdivided into mixed mesodermal tumours, in which heterologous elements, such as striated muscle and cartilage, can be found, and carcinosarcoma, in which such elements are not found. The term "sarcoma botryoides," often used for the polypoid form of such tumours, is best confined to the more truly grape-like tumours of younger patients, usually embryonal rhabdomyosarcomas.

Early references to müllerian mixed tumours were reviewed by Taylor (8) and Chuang et al. (1). The study discussed in this chapter was undertaken when an unusually large proportion of malignant tumours of the uterus in patients admitted to the Birmingham and Midland Hospital for Women was found to belong to this group. The best survival rates previously reported were 21% of 28 cases by Symmonds and Dockerty (6) and 42.4% of 33 cases by Taylor (8). We hoped that a review might shed some light as to why the müllerian mesoderm responded by tumour formation and hoped to obtain further information about the presentation and aetiology of the tumour.

PATIENTS AND CLINICAL FEATURES

In the period from 1972 through 1977, there were 28 cases of müllerian mixed tumours diagnosed and treated at the Birmingham and Midland Hospital for Women. During the same period, approximately 18,000 patients were admitted for gynaecological surgical procedures to the hospital, and of these, 213 were diagnosed and treated for adenocarcinoma of the corpus uteri.

The patients ranged between 48 and 83 years of age (mean 67.3 ± 12.4) at the time of initial presentation, and all but 1 patient were postmenopausal. The mean age of the menopause (49.3 ± 3.1 years) showed no difference from that expected in the normal population. Eight of the 28 patients (28.6%) were para 0, 15 were para 1 or 2, and 5 were para 3 or greater.

With the recent interest in the role of unopposed oestrogens and endometrial malignancies, this aspect was examined in our cases, but only 3 patients (10.7%) had ever received hormone replacement therapy at any time.

Of great interest and of possible aetiological relevance was the fact that 5 patients (17.8%) had had radium menopause induced 4 to 25 years prior to presentation, all for dysfunctional uterine bleeding problems. Another 5 patients had had diagnostic curettage, while 1 patient had a subtotal abdominal hysterectomy for the treatment of dysfunctional uterine haemorrhage in the perimenopausal period.

PRESENTING SYMPTOMS

The predominant presenting symptom (in 24 of 28 cases) was postmenopausal bleeding, with a history ranging between 1 and 6 months' duration. Vaginal discharge, metrorrhagia, urinary problems, or an abdominal mass were the symptoms in the remaining patients.

CYTOLOGY AND BIMANUAL EXAMINATION

Cervical and/or vault cytology had been performed in 21 patients. The smears were reported as follows: 9 positive with malignant cells of endometrial origin; 6 with atypical or suspicious glandular cells; 1 with atypical squamous cells; and 5 negative (grade I or II). However, even upon careful retrospective review of the slides, no specific cytological abnormalities differentiating these cases from endometrial adenocarcinoma were apparent.

The only significant findings upon bimanual examination in the patients were that in 18 cases the uterus was described as enlarged or bulky, and in another 4, an exophytic growth of the cervix was visible.

DIAGNOSIS AND MANAGEMENT

Definitive diagnosis of müllerian mixed tumour was made from uterine curettings in 20 patients, cervical biopsy in 3, vault biopsy in 1, and peritoneal biopsy in 1. In the remaining 3 patients, the curettings were initially reported as adenocarcinoma, and the true diagnosis was subsequently made on a section of the uterus.

The patients were managed by different consultant teams at the Birmingham and Midland Hospital for Women, and to date no standard treatment regime has been formalised. The most common procedure was the performance of a diagnostic curettage or cervical biopsy to establish the diagnosis, followed by total abdominal hysterectomy and bilateral salpingo-oophorectomy (16 cases). Five cases had dilation and curettage and intracavitary radium, followed by hysterectomy with bilateral salpingo-oophorectomy and node dissection, while in 3 cases, total abdominal hysterectomy and bilateral salpingo-oophorectomy were performed first, followed by postoperative vault radium.

FOLLOW-UP

Of the 28 patients studied in this series, only 7 remain alive; of these, 6 have survived for 5 years or more (5-year survival rate, 21.4%), and 1 has remained well after 4 years. Of the 21 nonsurvivors, 15 died within 12 months of initial diagnosis, 3 died in the second year, and 3 died more than 2 years after surgery. One patient died 2 days after surgery from a myocardial infarction.

Sixteen of the 28 patients showed evidence of spread beyond the uterus at the time of diagnosis. It is interesting to note that 1 patient had histological evidence of spread to the tubes and ovaries but remains alive and well 4 years after surgery, having received pelvic radiotherapy immediately after surgery.

Six patients with evidence of recurrence or widespread tumour at surgery were treated with pelvic radiotherapy or vault radium, and 4, with cytotoxic agents alone. Nine of these 10 patients were dead within 5 months after commencing treatment, and the tenth, within 8 months. Patients receiving these treatments did not seem to have improved survival rates in comparison with patients who did not receive such therapy.

DISCUSSION

In this series, over a 6-year period 1 case of müllerian mixed tumour was found for every 8 cases of adenocarcinoma of the corpus uteri; thus it would seem müllerian mixed tumours are not quite as rare as is commonly thought. Norris and Taylor (3) advocated the separation of müllerian mixed tumours into carcinosarcoma and mesodermal mixed tumour, since in their view carcinosarcoma had a better prognosis. In our view and others (1,7,9), there is no real difference between the two subgroups in terms of prognosis, and since the distinction between the two tumour groups is based only on the presence or absence of heterotopic elements, the recognition of which depends on many variable factors, the subclassification seems unhelpful.

The prognosis would seem to be directly related to whether or not the tumour is confined to the uterus at the time of surgical extirpation. Of the 21 nonsurvivors, 15 had clinical or microscopic evidence of spread beyond the uterus, 3 had deep tumour penetration of the myometrium, and 3 had only minimal myometrial invasion.

Our 5-year survival rate of 21.5% is comparable to that of many other series but is much less than the 42.2% reported by Taylor (9). However, of the 12 patients in whom the tumour appeared to be confined to the uterus at the time of diagnosis, a 50% 5-year survival rate was found, and a similar proportion of such patients in other series would be needed before results can be compared.

The question of whether or not the prior exposure of the uterine cavity to radiation predisposes to the development of müllerian mixed tumours is still disputed. Speert and Peightal (5) suggested that irradiation of the endometrium predisposed to the development of malignant disease, and Klein (2) quoted an incidence of previous irradiation in 11 of 29 cases of uterine carcinosarcoma. Chuang et al. (1) reported that 17% of cases with müllerian mixed tumour had received radiotherapy, but all were for other gynaecological malignancies.

In our series, 5 patients (17.8%) had received intracavitary radium for benign conditions to induce radiation menopause. In addition, 6 patients had received surgical treatment for dysfunctional uterine bleeding during the perimenopausal period. It is possible to postulate that it may not be the radium per se that results in the tumour process but rather it is the underlying cause of dysfunctional uterine haemorrhage.

In 14 of 20 uteri with residual endometrium, adenocarcinoma was found adjacent to the mixed müllerian area of the tumour, and in several cases these areas were quite extensive, sometimes associated with a squamous component. The finding of the 2 tumours in juxtaposition led Taylor (9) to postulate that malignant endometrial tumours may have a common müllerian histogenesis; in some, the sarcomatous component predominates, and in others, the carcinomatous component outgrows the other tissues.

The tumour is notoriously resistant to radiotherapy, and there would seem to be little benefit from the use of preoperative intracavitary radium or postoperative radiotherapy, except perhaps when the metastases are predominantly adenocarci-nomatous. In our series, chemotherapeutic agents were used only when secondary deposits were clinically obvious. Whether their use immediately postoperatively could have any effect on prognosis has yet to be assessed. At present, the only hope for long-term survival seems diagnosis and surgical removal early in the course of the disease.

SUMMARY

The salient clinical and histopathological features of 28 patients with müllerian mixed tumours of the uterine corpus presenting to the Birmingham and Midland Hospital for Women in the period from 1972 through 1977 were reviewed. The 5-year survival rate for this group was 21.4%, with 53.3% of the patients dying within 12 months of diagnosis. The most important finding of prognostic value was the extent of the tumour at the time of diagnosis, and where this was localised in the uterus, a 50% 5-year survival rate was found. The presence of specific types of heterotopic elements or numbers of mitotic figures was not correlated with the outcome. Five patients had previously received radium for the induction of radiation menopause, and the relevance of this treatment and other factors in the aetiology of the tumour was discussed.

REFERENCES

1. Chuang, J. T., Van Velden, D. J. J., and Graham, J. B. (1970): Carcinosarcoma and mixed mesodermal tumour of the uterine corpus. *Obstet. Gynecol.*, 35:769–780.
2. Klein, J. (1953): Carcinosarcoma of the endometrium. *Am. J. Obstet. Gynecol.*, 65:1212–1227.
3. Norris, H. J., and Taylor, H. B. (1966): Mesenchymal tumours of the uterus. III. A clinical and pathological study of 31 carcinosarcomas. *Cancer*, 19:1459–1465.
4. Poulsen, H. E., and Taylor, C. W. (editors) (1975): *International Histological Classification of Tumours, No. 15: Histological typing of the female genital tract tumours*, p. 69. World Health Organization, Geneva.

5. Speert, H., and Peightal, T. C. (1949): Malignant tumours of the uterine fundus subsequent to irradiation for benign pelvic conditions. *Am. J. Obstet. Gynecol.*, 57:261–273.
6. Symmonds, R. E., and Dockerty, M. B. (1955): Sarcoma and sarcoma-like proliferation of the endometrial stroma. I. A clinical study of 19 mesodermal mixed tumours. *Surg. Gynecol. Obstet.*, 100:232–240.
7. Symmonds, R. E., and Dockerty, M. B. (1955): Sarcoma and sarcoma-like proliferation of the endometrial stroma. II. Carcinosarcoma. *Surg. Gynecol. Obstet.*, 100:322–328.
8. Taylor, C. W. (1958): Mesodermal mixed tumours of the female genital tract. *J. Obstet. Gynaec. Brit. Emp.*, 65:177–188.
9. Taylor, C. W. (1972): Müllerian mixed tumours. *Acta Pathol. Microbiol. Scand.* (Suppl.), 233:48–55.

Recent Clinical Developments in Gynecologic Oncology, edited by C. Paul Morrow, et al.
Raven Press, New York © 1983.

Ovarian Tumors of Borderline Malignancy

H. Fox

Department of Pathology, Stopford Building, University of Manchester, Oxford Road, Manchester M13 9PT, England

A pathological report should represent a line of communication between the histopathologist and those directly concerned with the clinical care of the patient. However, this line is sometimes broken when a pathological report of ovarian tumor of borderline malignancy is issued, since there are a number of gynecologists who still believe that this diagnosis is indicative of indecision and that there are no borderline tumors but only borderline pathologists. If this were the case, then the gynecologist would have legitimate grounds for complaint, since little point would be served by elevating pathological indecisiveness to a nosological entity. However, this is not the case, since in pathological terms tumors of borderline malignancy form a well-delineated and well-defined group of ovarian neoplasms, the diagnosis of which is a positive one based on specific histological features. It is true that the pathologist is using a term that hints at uncertainty and irresolution, but the term "borderline malignancy" does correctly describe the biological status of these tumors, which are neither fully benign nor overtly malignant but occupy a gray hinterland between these two extremes of orderly, controlled proliferation and cellular anarchy.

A number of alternative names do, of course, exist for these tumors. Some refer to them by the term "tumors of low-grade malignancy," but this expression is often applied to neoplasms in other parts of the body that are clearly, although indolently, malignant and implies that all borderline tumors are inherently malignant, an implication that may or may not be true. Others use "carcinomas of low malignant potential," but this term has the dual drawbacks of being relatively meaningless in biological terms and of indicating the essentially carcinomatous nature of all borderline neoplasms. The term "proliferating epithelial tumors" has its adherents, but all tumors, benign or malignant, consist of proliferating cells and hence this expression is too all embracing.

DEFINITION

The Panel on Nomenclature of Ovarian Tumours of the World Health Organization (WHO) (19) has defined a borderline tumor as "one that has some, but not all, of the morphological features of malignancy; those present include in varying combinations: stratification of epithelial cells, apparent detachment of cellular clusters from their sites of origin and mitotic figures and nuclear abnormalities intermediate between those of clearly benign and unquestionably malignant tumours of a similar cell type; on the other hand, obvious invasion of the adjacent stroma is lacking." It should be noted that this definition is based solely on the histological features of the ovarian tumor and does not take into account whether or not there is extraovarian spread, a fact that sometimes disconcerts gynecologists who are informed that an ovarian neoplasm that is clinically stage 2 or 3 is one that is histologically only of borderline malignancy.

The WHO definition has several obvious drawbacks: it does not elaborate on the degree of mitotic activity and nuclear abnormality, which can be classed as "intermediate" between benign and malignant tumors, does not indicate in precise terms what is meant by "obvious" stromal invasion, and does not sufficiently stress that lack of stromal invasion is of prime diagnostic importance. This last deficiency has been exploited, quite reasonably, by some who maintain that a neoplasm, particularly one of mucinous type, in which there are very marked epithelial abnormalities can be classed as an adenocarcinoma even in the absence of obvious stromal invasion (5,6). This attitude is, to some extent, based on the difficulty that may be encountered, especially in mucinous tumors, in deciding whether stromal invasion is absent or not, and in recent years there has been a subtle alteration in the WHO definition of a borderline tumor insofar as there has been a tendency to insist not on a lack of obvious stromal invasion but on the absence of destructive stromal invasion. Unfortunately, the term "destructive" in this context has not always been clearly defined, and there is no doubt that in many nonovarian tumors, stromal invasion can occur without any tissue destruction or reaction.

At St. Mary's Hospital in Manchester, England, it has been our practice to consider a tumor of borderline malignancy as one in which the epithelium shows some or all of the characteristics of malignancy but in which there is no stromal invasion. It will be recognized that this particular working definition does not take into account the degree of severity of the epithelial abnormalities and in this respect departs somewhat from the WHO definition and considerably from those who are prepared to diagnose an adenocarcinoma even in the absence of stromal invasion. The insistence on the lack of stromal invasion as a defining feature does not take into account whether the invasion is destructive or not, and extensive sampling, coupled with a readiness to resort to serial sectioning, is clearly necessary to establish a negative finding of this type. However, it is readily admitted that it is often difficult and sometimes almost impossible to determine whether stromal invasion is present or absent. If even after extensive examination doubt with respect to this remains, it seems reasonable to transmit this fact in the pathological report and to advise that tumors with questionable stromal invasion should probably best be regarded as adenocarcinomas.

INCIDENCE

The borderline tumors form a significant proportion of the overall group of epithelial ovarian neoplasms. In Russell's series (15,16) from Sydney, Australia, of 1,000 ovarian epithelial neoplasms, 11.4% were classed as neoplams of borderline malignancy, while in the Manchester Ovarian Tumour Registry (which registers all ovarian tumors seen in five hospitals), there were, in the five-year period 1974–1979, 778 epithelial neoplasms, of which 9.9% fell into the borderline malignancy category. In the Manchester series, 7.6% of the serous tumors were of borderline malignancy, while 19% of the mucinous tumors fell into this category. Expressing the figures differently, 24% of all nonbenign serous tumors in the Manchester series were of borderline malignancy, as were 44% of all nonbenign mucinous tumors; the comparable figures in Russell's (16) series were 23.6% for serous tumors and 75% for mucinous tumors. It is interesting to note that our figures for the serous neoplasms tally exactly with Russell's but that there is a wide disparity between the two series in the figures for mucinous tumors. Russell's incidence of borderline mucinous tumors is close to that found by Hart and Norris (6), while the incidence in our series is in close accord with that in a number of other studies in which 37 to 52% of all nonbenign mucinous tumors were classed as borderline (1,11,17).

PATHOLOGY

It is generally maintained, with considerable truth, that there is a continuous spectrum of appearances between fully benign and frankly malignant ovarian neoplasms, and it is often thought that tumors of borderline malignancy occupy the middle part of this spectral range. However, the gross morphology of borderline tumors lies closer to the benign than the malignant extreme of this spectrum, and the combined gross and histological appearances of most borderline tumors are sufficiently characteristic to allow for their ready recognition.

Nearly all borderline tumors are of either the serous or mucinous variety. Borderline forms of the other epithelial ovarian neoplasms do exist, but are all rare with the possible exception of the endometrioid type.

Serous Tumors of Borderline Malignancy

Serous tumors of borderline malignancy are nearly always papillary and macroscopically most resemble benign papillary serous cystadenomas. A distinction from a fully benign tumor is sometimes possible with the naked eye on the basis of a more luxuriant proliferation of fine papillae and the presence of exophytic papillary excrescences on the outer surface of the cyst. A small proportion of borderline serous tumors are grossly similar to benign papillary serous surface tumors but tend to have a more complex and dense papillary pattern. Histologically, the borderline serous tumors are formed of rather fine branching papillae with fibrous cores (Fig. 1). The cellular mantle of the papillae can be clearly recognized in tumors with minimal epithelial irregularity as being of the tubal type, but in tumors with marked epithelial abnormalities, this tubal pattern is lost and the cells have a rather uniform rounded or cuboid appearance. The epithelial component of the tumors (Fig. 2) shows a variable degree of multilayering and has a marked tendency to form cellular buds or tufts. These buds may break off to float freely within the cyst lumen, while fusion, or coalescence, of the tips of adjacent epithelial buds may give rise to a somewhat honeycombed pattern. Nuclear crowding, atypia, and hyperchromatism

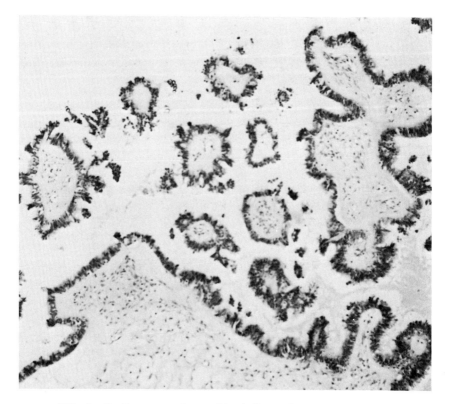

FIG. 1. Papillary serous tumor of borderline malignancy (H. & E. ×60).

are of variable degree, but the nucleoli are not often particularly prominent. Mitotic figures are rather uncommon and rarely of atypical form. Psammoma bodies are frequently present and are of no diagnostic significance. In most borderline serous tumors, there is a sharp junction between epithelium and stroma, and the possibility of stromal invasion can be excluded with relative ease. In others, there may be epithelial invaginations into the stroma, and these can cause diagnostic difficulty, which, however, is often resolved by serial sectioning. By and large, all borderline serous tumors have a strikingly similar appearance and present an easily recognizable and characteristic histological pattern. Furthermore, the borderline pattern of epithelial abnormality is relatively constant throughout these neoplasms, and it is most unusual to find areas of clearly benign epithelium alternating or intermingling with epithelium that has malignant characteristics.

A notable feature of borderline serous tumors is the high incidence of bilaterality, variously estimated as being between 14 and 33% (8,13). The bilateral involvement is not always apparent to the naked eye and may be only recognized upon histological examination. However, it is almost certain that the bilaterality is due to the con-current development of two independent primary tumors rather than to metastasis

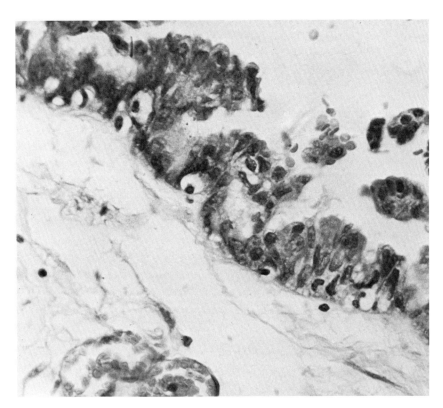

FIG. 2. Epithelium in papillary serous tumor of borderline malignancy. Multilayering and budding is present, some cellular buds having detached from epithelium (H. & E. ×300).

of a single primary lesion to the contralateral ovary. A further and often disconcerting aspect of borderline neoplasms is the frequency of apparent extraovarian spread at the time of initial diagnosis, which usually takes the form of multiple seedlings or implants on the pelvic peritoneum and the omentum. The presence of such implants has been noted in 16 to 47% of cases (8,13,16), and the fact that they are sometimes accompanied by ascites often provokes a gloomy prognostic attitude. However, histological examination shows that many of these implants are deep within rather than on the surface of the peritoneum and that some have a benign appearance and do not show any invasive tendencies. Most will show a borderline pattern, and it is relatively uncommon for there to be an overtly carcinomatous picture. Some peritoneal implants do progress in a rather indolent and leisurely fashion, but many either remain stationary for many years or regress (3). There are good grounds for believing that most are not true implants or metastases but represent multiple foci of neoplastic transformation, not necessarily or even usually of a malignant nature, within peritoneal mesothelium (16); indeed, in many instances, the condition can be classed as a form of endosalpingiosis.

Mucinous Tumors of Borderline Malignancy

Mucinous tumors of borderline malignancy usually present as large multilocular cysts. The outer lining of the cyst is smooth, but focal areas of thickening, nodularity, or endophytic papillary projections should alert the pathologist to the possibility of a borderline rather than benign tumor. Borderline mucinous tumors differ significantly from their serous counterparts in that there is no uniformity of appearance throughout the neoplasm; some areas have a fully benign epithelial pattern, while others show a variable degree of epithelial irregularity and abnormality. The areas of borderline malignancy may be extremely focal, and hence all mucinous tumors need to be extensively sampled. In borderline mucinous tumors, the epithelium may show a complex glandular pattern (Fig. 3) but is often characterized by short papillary infoldings (Fig. 4), which give the epithelium a serrated appearance. There are varying degrees of multilayering, loss of polarity, nuclear hyperchromatism, and cellular atypia, while mitotic figures tend to be seen with some frequency, albeit usually of normal form. Because of the outpouching of the

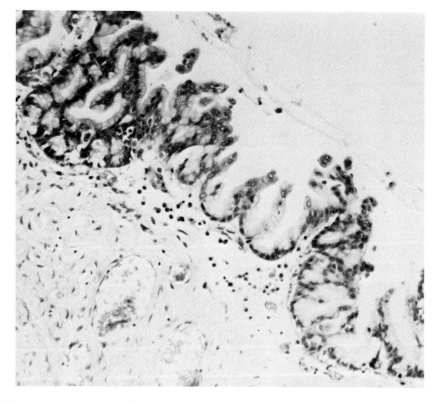

FIG. 3. Mucinous tumor of borderline malignancy. Complex multiglandular pattern above and to left (H. & E. ×120).

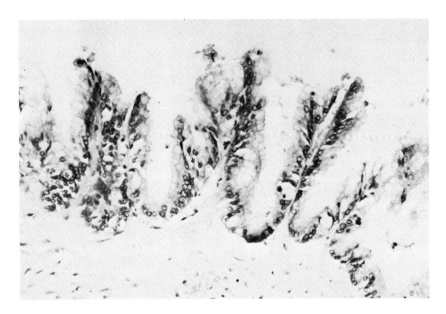

FIG. 4. Mucinous tumor of borderline malignancy. Epithelium shows papillary pattern (H. & E. ×120).

epithelium and the formation of secondary cysts or glands in many borderline mucinous tumors, the assessment of possible stromal invasion is more difficult than in the case of serous tumors. However, Russell (16) has pointed out that this is not usually an impossible task, since features such as an irregular contour and arrangement of the glandular structures, a focal chronic inflammatory cell reaction, and the presence of immature-type stroma all suggest invasion rather than inclusion. Certainly there can be no doubt that invasion is occurring if single cells, nests of cells, or cellular cords are seen infiltrating the stroma. Nevertheless, Hart and Norris (6) have maintained that, in the absence of definite stromal invasion, a mucinous tumor should be regarded as malignant rather than borderline if there is marked overgrowth of atypical epithelial cells or striking nuclear abnormalities. They also suggest that finger-like papillary projections of solid cellular masses without a stromal support should be regarded as diagnostic of adenocarcinoma and view as malignant those borderline tumors in which stratification of atypical epithelial cells has exceeded three layers in thickness. Russell (16) has commented that "these supplementary criteria seem to add an unnecessary complication to an already difficult area which is not justified by an increased precision of prognosis." His is a sentiment that our experience at St. Mary's Hospital would lead us to endorse.

Borderline mucinous tumors are much less commonly bilateral than borderline serous tumors. In Hart and Norris' series (6) approximately 10% of the borderline mucinous tumors were bilateral, while in Russell's series of 52 cases, none were bilateral (16). Our own experience would suggest a figure somewhere between these two. Although Aure et al. (1) found that about 15% of ovarian borderline neoplasms had extended beyond the confines of the ovary at the time of diagnosis, it would be the experience of most, and certainly our own, that such extraovarian spread is very much less common than this figure would suggest. Certainly, the picture of widespread peritoneal and omental implants is rarely seen with mucinous borderline tumors. However, a relatively common feature of these neoplasms is pseudomyxoma ovarii, which was encountered in 25% of Russell's cases (16). This condition, which is due to the leakage of mucus into the ovarian stromal tissues, sometimes provokes a pseudosarcomatous reaction in the stromal tissue and progresses to pseudomyxoma peritoneii in about 50% of cases.

Borderline Endometrioid Tumors

Borderline endometrioid tumors are generally thought of as rare (1,17), although in Russell's series, 18% of all endometrioid neoplasms were of the borderline variety (16). In the Manchester 1974–79 series, there were no borderline endometrioid tumors, but it has been our experience that at St. Mary's Hospital there has been an increase in the number of such neoplasms in the past few years. Such borderline tumors are almost invariably seen in association with and apparently arising from foci of ovarian endometriosis, and the histological appearances greatly resemble those of an atypical hyperplasia of the endometrium (Fig. 5). Indeed, it is a moot point as to whether lesions of this type should be regarded as neoplastic or hyperplastic, and all the difficulties that are encountered in differentiating between a severe atypical hyperplasia and an adenocarcinoma in the endometrium find their exact counterpart in these ovarian lesions. We and others (9) have seen a small number of endometrioid adenofibromas of borderline malignancy in which endometrial-type glands showing irregular budding, stratification, and nuclear atypia are set in an abundant, dense fibrous stroma.

Brenner Tumors of Borderline Malignancy

Brenner tumors of borderline malignancy form a clear-cut entity (4,12,14). Such neoplasms are usually unilateral and rather large. They are wholly or partly cystic, and their cut surface shows multiple locules containing watery or mucoid fluid. In some areas, the locular lining is smooth, but in others it is formed by papillary, velvety, friable tissue that grows into the cyst lumen. Histologically, areas of typical benign Brenner tumor are often but not invariably present, while in the papillary areas of the tumor, the epithelium forms multilayered folds supported by thin connective tissue stalks. The appearances in these areas bear an uncanny and unmistakable resemblance to those of a grade 1 transitional cell carcinoma of the bladder (Fig. 6). Focal cellular atypia and nuclear atypia are usually present, and there is often a sprinkling of mitotic figures. Stromal invasion, which is easy to assess in these neoplasms, is not seen.

Mesonephroid Tumors of Borderline Malignancy

In our experience and that of others (10), mesonephroid tumors of borderline malignancy always appear to take the form of a mesonephroid (or "clear-cell")

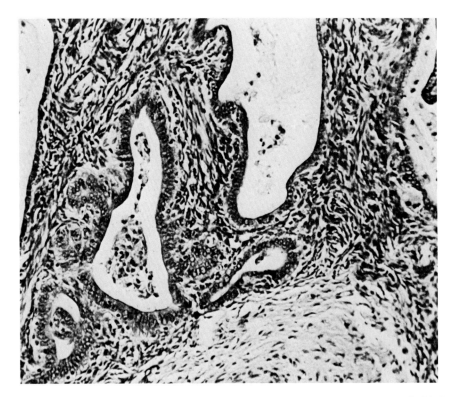

FIG. 5. Endometrioid tumor of borderline malignancy, seen in focus of endometriosis (H. & E. ×120).

adenofibroma, in which epithelial glands lined by hob-nail or clear cells showing varying degrees of cellular and nuclear atypia are embedded in a fibrous stroma.

CLINICAL FEATURES

The histological specificity of the borderline group of neoplasms is not accompanied by any atypical, or diagnostic, clinical features. The only exception to this rule is that borderline serous tumors often occur in relatively young women, aged 30 to 40, and hence the presence of an ovarian neoplasm in a woman of this age, especially if there is bilateral involvement or if accompanied by ascites, should arouse a strong suspicion of a borderline epithelial tumor.

PROGNOSIS

There is some doubt with respect to the long-term prognosis for women with a tumor of borderline malignancy. There is, of course, general agreement that the prognosis is good for most patients, certainly in the short term, but there has been some disagreement about the long-term prognosis. There is a consensus that the 5-year survival rate of patients with a serous tumor of borderline malignancy is in

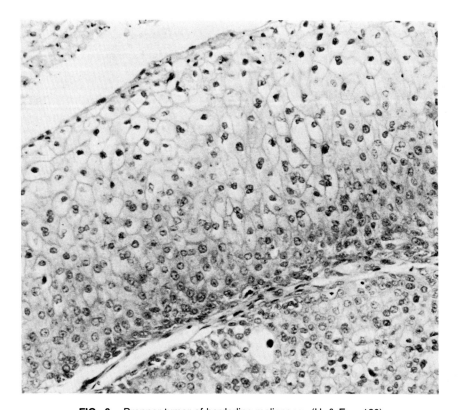

FIG. 6. Brenner tumor of borderline malignancy (H. & E. × 120).

the vicinity of 90% (1,8,13), but reported 10-year survival rates have varied from 75 to 90% (1,8,17). It should be stressed that these survival rates are virtually independent both of the clinical stage of the neoplasm and the presence of residual tumor; patients with extraovarian spread or residual tumor appear to have a prognosis very little worse than that for women with neoplasms confined to the ovary and with no obvious residual disease. The 5-year survival rate for women with borderline mucinous tumors is extremely good, probably in the vicinity of 95% (6), but estimates of the 10-year survival rate have ranged from 68 to 95% (1,6,17).

PROGNOSTIC INDICATORS

It is clear that although the overall prognosis for women with borderline ovarian tumors is good, a small number will die as a direct result of their ovarian neoplasm. A high 5- or 10-year survival rate may appear initially reassuring to a woman with such a tumor, but human beings are less concerned with the overall survival of the diagnostic group to which they belong than they are with their own individual chances of survival. The problem of formulating an individual prognosis or at least of giving a clearer indication of the likelihood of a particular patient being one of the unfortunate minority who succumb to their disease is a challenging one. This challenge is posed principally to the pathologist, since in this group of neoplasms the gynecologist is deprived of the most important clinical prognostic indicator, namely, staging, and hence has to rely on some other form of assessment, such as tumor grading.

The concept of borderline neoplasms encompasses tumors with a wide range of epithelial abnormalities, ranging from tumors in which there is only a minimal deviation from a fully benign pattern to those distinguished from a frank adenocarcinoma only by the absence of stromal invasion. It therefore would appear logical to suggest that tumors in which the epithelial abnormalities are at the malignant end of the spectrum would be more likely to have a poorer long-term prognosis than those at the benign end and that tumor grading therefore would be of prognostic value. Russell (16) has introduced a grading system for borderline tumors in which 4 particular features are assessed: epithelial budding, epithelial multilayering, mitotic activity, and nuclear atypia. Each of these features is given a grade ranging from 1 for minor degrees of abnormality to 4 for severe abnormality. Russell found that in the borderline serous tumors, grading was achieved most easily by an assessment of the degree of epithelial budding and showed that while 91.6% of the tumors in grade 1 were clinically stage 1, only 78% of grade 2 tumors exhibited no extraovarian spread. Furthermore, only 30.5% of the grade 1 and 2 tumors were bilateral, while both ovaries were involved in 54.5% of grade 3 and 4 neoplasms. These figures could be taken either as indicating a correlation between histological grade and the degree of local aggressiveness or as showing that the more actively proliferating tumors are associated with a more widespread multifocal neoplastic process.

Russell did not indicate if there was a correlation between histological grade and long-term prognosis. However, if grading of borderline tumors is to be of value, two conditions must be met: (a) the grading system should be one that can be applied in a consistent manner, and (b) the grading system must have some prognostic value.

At St. Mary's Hospital, we have recently tested the ease and consistency with which borderline ovarian tumors can be graded. Three pathologists, all working in the same laboratory and all with a particular interest in ovarian neoplasms, were asked to grade independently 37 tumors that all 3 agreed were of borderline malignancy. Only a single representative slide from each tumor was examined, and the pathologists were all to apply the same criteria. The grading was based on an assessment of the same 4 epithelial abnormalities used in Russell's study, but only 3 grades were specified: benign end of spectrum, malignant end of spectrum, and intermediate. In only 43% of the tumors did all 3 pathologists allot the same grade. They fared somewhat better with the serous tumors, being in agreement in 47% of cases, than they did with the mucinous tumors, in which agreement was achieved in only 36%. In most cases in which there was disagreement about the grade, 2 of the pathologists (not necessarily the same 2 in each instance) differed from the third, but in 14% of cases, a different grade was allotted to the same tumor by each of the 3 pathologists. It seems not unreasonable to conclude from this exercise that histological grading of borderline ovarian tumors tends to be highly subjective and that it is difficult to apply a grading system in a consistent and generally applicable manner. It is possible that these difficulties could be overcome by the use of computer-aided quantitative histological techniques of the type that have recently been applied to the study of mucinous tumors (2). However, such techniques are extremely time consuming, and their introduction into routine use could only be justified if histological grading of these tumors was clearly shown to be of prognostic value. Unfortunately, our own experience suggests that it may be difficult to establish the value of histological grading. A 5-year follow-up was made of the 37 patients whose borderline tumors had been the subject of the attempted grading. Only 24 of the patients could be traced, and of these, 20 were alive and well, the remaining 4 having died as a result of their ovarian tumor. In the 4 fatal cases, all 3 pathologists agreed that 3 of the tumors were either at the benign end or in the middle of the spectrum of malignancy. The fourth tumor was thought to be at the malignant end of the spectrum by 2 pathologists and in the middle of the range by the third. Conversely, there were a few cases in which all 3 pathologists agreed that the tumor was at the benign end of the spectrum, and in all these cases the patient was alive and well, as were all patients in whom an agreed grading at the malignant end of the spectrum was achieved. These findings have resulted in some disillusionment about the value of histological grading of borderline tumors.

Another approach to the grading of borderline tumors is the quantitative immunohistological assessment of their content of secretory products. Heald et al. (7) found that many ovarian epithelial tumors, whether benign or malignant, contained carcinoembryonic antigen (CEA), and while semiquantitative measurement of the tumor content of CEA using a dilutional technique failed to reveal any discriminatory differences between benign and serous neoplasms, there was a clear-cut difference between malignant mucinous tumors, which invariably had a high content of CEA, and benign mucinous neoplasms, which either had a low content of or stained negatively for CEA. A measurement of the CEA content of borderline mucinous tumors showed that about 50% had a CEA content similar to that of malignant tumors, while the remainder had a CEA content more typical of a benign neoplasm. In the borderline group of neoplasms, there was no relationship between the CEA content and the degree of epithelial abnormality, but it could be postulated that borderline neoplasms with a high CEA content may be more likely to pursue a malignant course than those with low CEA levels. Unfortunately, it still remains to be proven that this is indeed the case.

MANAGEMENT OF BORDERLINE TUMORS

It is clearly difficult to suggest hard and fast rules for the management of borderline ovarian neoplasms. It is usually advised that in older women the optimal treatment of a tumor of borderline malignancy is hysterectomy and bilateral salpingo-oophorectomy. This is also probably the treatment of choice for patients of all ages with bilateral borderline tumors. However, in younger women who wish to preserve their reproductive capacity, it is probably justifiable if the tumor is stage 1a and if biopsy shows no involvement of the contralateral ovary to perform a unilateral salpingo-oophorectomy. Many would suggest that removal of the contralateral adnexa and the uterus should be undertaken in such patients after they have completed their families. A difficult problem arises in the management of serous borderline tumors with peritoneal implants. Scully's suggestion (18) that therapy in such cases should be based on the degree of differentiation and extent of the implants seems eminently sensible. If the implants appear histologically malignant, then the patient should probably be treated as a stage 2 carcinoma, and if the implants have a benign appearance, they probably can be safely ignored. It remains uncertain as to what the proper therapeutic approach should be if the implants have a borderline appearance, but it is probable that conservative treatment is justified in most cases.

CONCLUSION

A review of ovarian tumors of borderline malignancy clearly indicates that such tumors are now a well-established group that should be fully accepted in both histological and clinical terms. Unfortunately, the recognition of these tumors poses more questions than it answers, some of a basic biological nature and others of practical importance. These include the following:

1. Are borderline tumors benign neoplasms that are undergoing malignant change, or have they been of borderline type *ab initio*?

2. Do all borderline tumors eventually become overtly malignant?

3. Can borderline tumors remain confined to the ovary *ad infinitum*, or do they all eventually spread?

4. In mucinous tumors, in which multiple foci of borderline pattern alternate with benign epithelium, is there polyclonal malignant change?

5. Should mucinous tumors with severe epithelial atypia be classed as malignant even in the absence of stromal invasion?

6. What is the long-term prognosis for patients with borderline tumors?

7. What is the correct management of borderline serous tumors with extraovarian spread?

8. Can borderline serous tumors without extraovarian spread be safely treated by unilateral salpingo-oophorectomy, or is hysterectomy and bilateral salpingo-oophorectomy necessary?

9. Is it ethical to set up clinical controlled trials of the various forms of surgical therapy for borderline tumors?

No doubt the answers to these questions will be forthcoming in the future, but currently they remain a challenge to both pathologists and gynecologists.

REFERENCES

1. Aure, J. C., Hoeg, K., and Kolstad, P. (1971): Clinical and histological studies of ovarian carcinoma: Long term follow-up of 990 cases. *Obstet. Gynecol.*, 37:1–9.
2. Baak, J. P. A., Agrafojo, B. A., Kurver, P. H. J., Langley, F. A., Boon, M. E., Lindeman, J., Overdiep, S. H., Niouwlatt, A., and Brekelmans, E. (1981): Quantitation of borderline and malignant mucinous ovarian tumors. *Histopathology*, 5:353–360.

3. Fox, H., and Langley, F. A. (1976): *Tumours of the Ovary*. William Heinemann, London.
4. Hallgrimson, J., and Scully, R. E. (1972): Borderline and malignant Brenner tumors of the ovary: A report of 15 cases. *Acta Pathol. Microbiol. Scand. [A]* (Suppl. 233), 80:56–66.
5. Hart, W. R. (1977): Ovarian epithelial tumors of borderline malignancy (carcinoma of low malignant potential). *Hum. Pathol.*, 8:541–549.
6. Hart, W. R., and Norris, H. J. (1973): Borderline and malignant mucinous tumors of the ovary: Histologic criteria and clinical behaviour. *Cancer*, 31:1031–1045.
7. Heald, J., Buckley, C. H., and Fox, H. (1979): An immunohistochemical study of the distribution of carcinoembryonic antigen in epithelial tumours of the ovary. *J. Clin. Pathol.*, 32:919–926.
8. Julian, C. G., and Woodruff, J. D. (1972): The biological behaviour of low-grade papillary serous carcinoma of the ovary. *Obstet. Gynecol.*, 40:860–867.
9. Kao, G. F., and Norris, H. J. (1978): Cystadenofibroma of the ovary with epithelial atypism. *Amer J. Surg. Pathol.*, 2:357–363.
10. Kao, G. F., and Norris, H. J. (1979): Unusual cystadenofibromas: endometrioid, mucinous, and clear cell types. *Obstet. Gynecol.*, 54:729–736.
11. Luisi, I. (1968): Malignant ovarian tumors of Mullerian origin: some aspects. In: *Ovarian Cancer: U.I.C.C. Monograph Series, Volume II*, edited by J. Gentil and A. C. Junquiera, pp. 9–22. Springer-Verlag, Berlin.
12. Miles, P. A., and Norris, H. J. (1972): Proliferative and malignant Brenner tumors of the ovary. *Cancer*, 30:174–186.
13. Purola, E. (1963): Serous papillary ovarian tumours: A study of 233 cases with special reference to histological type of tumour and its influence on prognosis. *Acta Obstet Gynecol. Scand.*, [Suppl.], 42.
14. Roth, L. M., and Sternberg, W. H. (1971): Proliferating Brenner tumors. *Cancer*, 27:687–693.
15. Russell, P. (1979): The pathological assessment of ovarian neoplasms. I. Introduction to the common "epithelial" tumours and analysis of benign "epithelial" tumours. *Pathology*, 11:5–26.
16. Russell, P. (1979): The pathological assessment of ovarian neoplasms. II. The proliferating "epithelial" tumours. *Pathology*, 11:251–282.
17. Santesson, I., and Kottmeier, H. L. (1968): General classification of ovarian tumors. In: *Ovarian Cancer: U.I.C.C. Monograph Series, Volume II*, edited by J. Gentil and A. C. Junquiera, pp. 1–8. Springer-Verlag, Berlin.
18. Scully, R. E. (1979): *Atlas of Tumor Pathology, Second Series, Fasc. 16: Tumors of the Ovary and Maldeveloped Gonads*. Armed Forces Institute of Pathology, Washington, D.C.
19. Serov, S. F., Scully, R. E., and Sobin, L. H. (1973): *International Histological Classification of Tumours No. 9: Histological Typing of Ovarian Tumours*. World Health Organization, Geneva.

Recent Clinical Developments in Gynecologic Oncology, edited by C. Paul Morrow, et al.
Raven Press, New York © 1983.

Chemotherapy of Ovarian Carcinoma

J. J. Fennelly

*St. Vincent's Hospital and National Maternity Hospital,
Elm Park, Dublin, Ireland*

It has often been said that for ovarian cancer seemingly everything works but practically nothing succeeds. This is a reasonable statement, since having treated more than 150 patients with ovarian cancer over the last 10 years, I have seen that the initial surgery can often appear to be quite successful, radiation may prove to be of value, and chemotherapy can produce good results, although in most cases these measures prove to be of a temporary nature. For 20 years we have known of the good response to alkylating-agent therapy, but the ultimate effect on survival has remained small. In reading papers on ovarian cancer, the bias of results of treatment and the type of treatment often depend on the specialty of the research, e.g., gynaecology, radiotherapy, or medical oncology.

The major problem with ovarian carcinoma is that in most cases the disease is at an advanced stage at the time of diagnosis—60% of cases present primarily with stage III or IV disease. Great difficulty has long been encountered in initial and posttreatment evaluation, but the recent introduction of ultrasound, CT scan, laparoscopy, and second-look laparotomy have helped in proper and accurate staging and response to treatment. The rapid development of resistance to alkylating agents has been a major problem, and consequently combination chemotherapy would now appear to be the best form of chemotherapy in ovarian carcinoma. If we examine the relationship between stage and prognosis, as outlined by Tobias and Griffiths (15), we see that in stage I cases, i.e., very early disease, the survival rate is still relatively low, up to 65%, although some series have found a 5-year survival rate of 75 to 80%. When the disease is more advanced within the pelvis (stage II), the survival rate is 40 to 50%. The problem with stage III disease is that we are dealing with a variety of groups, ranging from patients with microscopic disease, which is not really measurable, to those with gross abdominal disease. Obviously there is considerable disparity in the survival rate between these two groups, and one would seek to bring about a cure in patients with early stage III disease, something that is probably not possible in patients with advanced stage III disease.

A number of factors have contributed to a changing outlook, some of which are outlined in Table 1.

TABLE 1. *Factors contributing to changing outlook in ovarian carcinoma*

Adequate evaluation
CT scan
Ultrasound
Laparoscopy
Detailed trials
Bush (4)
Young (18)
Wiltshawe (17)
Cis-platinum
Adjuvant therapy
Possible second-look evaluation

ALKYLATING AGENTS IN OVARIAN CARCINOMA

An examination of the major studies, with a combined total of 300 to 500 cases, reveals that the responses level out at about 50% regardless of whether one uses melphalan, cyclophosphamide, chlorambucil, thio-TEPA (19), or the more recently introduced treosulfan (7).

Treosulfan (dihydroxybusulfan) is an alkylating agent that acts as a diepoxide rather than a methanesulphone. In the author's experience, it is very well tolerated, causes minimal gastrointestinal toxicity and transient marrow depression in short-term usage, and is as effective as the other available alkylating agents. The use of such agents has long contributed to responses usually lasting about 8 to 12 months, whereupon total resistance developed.

Of the nonalkylating agents, *cis*-platinum has proven to be the most effective, in most series producing a response rate of about 50%.

Upon examining clinical trials of other agents, such as hexamethylmelamine, adriamycin, methotrexate, and 5-fluorouracil, it is found that most were used in cases that were resistant to alkylating agents, and consequently the disease continued to progress and the prognosis was poor.

STAGE I DISEASE

The exact role of adjuvant therapy in patients with stage I disease still remains unclear. Hreshchyshyn (8) compared stage I patients with ovarian cancer who had undergone surgery to patients who had radiotherapy following surgery (5,000 rads total pelvis) and patients who received melphalan following the primary surgical treatment. After 5 years, he noted a 6% recurrence rate in those receiving chemotherapy compared to 30% in those who received radiation treatment and 17% in those who did not. This would suggest that chemotherapy has some importance in disease management, and this factor has been utilized in single-agent therapy. Further studies are still needed with proper comparison with radiation therapy; in addition, the role of combination chemotherapy should be examined using *cis*-platinum in the combination. It is essential to exclude from such studies patients with very good prognostic histology (5).

ACUTE LEUKAEMIA IN OVARIAN CANCER

It would now be useful to mention the hazards of alkylating agents. In patients who have undergone long-term treatment of malignancies, such as patients with Hodgkin's disease, myeloma, and ovarian and breast cancer, there has been a definite increased incidence of acute leukaemia. Bush, in his excellent book on the management of ovarian carcinoma (4) described a risk ratio of 170/1; a similar ratio, 171/4, was noted by Reimer et al. (13), while Pedersen-Bjergaard (12) mentioned a ratio of 176/1 with the use of Treosulfan. All the patients in these studies had been on long-term alkylating agents, and all had long survival rates. This factor must affect one's approach to patients with early disease who may do well anyway, and therefore patients with localised disease with highly differentiated tumours could advisedly receive no adjuvant treatment, since their outlook is so good (5).

STAGE II DISEASE

There are many reports on the use of radiotherapy after surgery in stage II disease, most suggesting benefits from the treatments. Upon examining the results of various authors, such as Van Orden et al. (16), Barr et al. (3), and Kent and McKay (9), it indeed appears that patients who received radiation after surgery had better survival rates; however, these were not prospectively controlled trials. At present, the question as to whether radiation or chemotherapy should be used as an adjuvant in Stage II disease remains unclear. This author favours the use of combination chemotherapy, with a full review of the patient at 6 to 12 months.

STAGE III DISEASE

It is essential to subdivide stage III according to the volume of residual disease, since it is clear that patients who have minimal residual disease may be quite responsive to irradiation, whereas those with bulky residual disease will not respond and chemotherapy would appear to be the principal mode of management. Bush (4) has shown that in patients with stage III disease who have minimal residual disease, the use of strip irradiation can be successful, providing good long-term results with tolerable side effects. However, for patients with more advanced disease, chemotherapy would appear to be the primary mode of management. With the knowledge that a single alkylating agent produces response rates in about 50% of cases for relatively brief periods of time and knowing the benefits of *cis*-platinum, it does appear logical to combine the two. One of the best results to date is that reported by Barker and Wiltshawe (2), who achieved a 52% response rate, with 25% complete responses in patients treated with chlorambucil and *cis*-platinum; the addition of adriamycin proved of little benefit. The median duration of those with complete response was 31 months. Barker and Wiltshawe concluded that "for optimal results in ovarian carcinoma total tumours ridded within 6 to 12 months by either drugs alone or in combination with cytoreductive surgery would appear to be the only chance of prolonged survival." Many additional trials are needed before this can be evaluated fully. In a controlled clinical trial comparing melphalan with Hexa-CAF (hexamethylmelamine, cyclophosphamide, methotrexate, 5-fluorouracil), Young and others (1,18) of the National Cancer Institute demonstrated that Hexa-CAF produced a 75% response, compared to a 50% response obtained with the use of melphalan alone. The duration of the response to the combination therapy was much longer; however, toxicity proved to be quite high with the combination therapy and minimal with the single agent. In patients with advanced and presumably incurable disease, serious thought should be given to the question of using highly toxic regimens.

STAGE IV DISEASE

In stage IV disease, cytotoxic therapy obviously plays a major role, and only in the presence of local symptoms is irradiation of real benefit. It is important that one be aware of the toxicity of the drugs used and be certain that treatment is indeed beneficial. Most studies describe responses of about 50% lasting 6 to 18 months (7,17) using single alkylating agents, with higher responses, e.g., 75% (18) and 83% (11), occurring with combination chemotherapy. Great care should be taken that real benefit is being achieved in the incurable patient undergoing combination therapy, which produces a higher number of side effects.

OTHER TUMOURS

Various types of germ-cell tumours occur in ovarian malignancy, of which dys-germinoma and yolk-sac tumours are the most common. Dysgerminoma is usually managed by surgery but has a tendency to spread to the lymph nodes. Consequently, lymphangiography plays a certain role in the staging of the disease, since if the nodes are affected, radiation would prove beneficial because such tumours are highly radiosensitive. Yolk-sac tumours occur primarily in the paediatric age group, are highly malignant, spread rapidly through the abdomen, and are not sensitive to radiation.

Smith and Rutledge (14) have reported obtaining good results with chemotherapy using a combination of three drugs: vincristine, actinomycin D, and cyclophos-phamide (VAC). This has not been the case at our hospital, where we have used a programme similar to that mentioned by Lokey et al. (10). In my experience, in 3 patients on VAC therapy, the results have been poor. More recently, using therapy similar to that used in testicular germ-cell tumours, i.e., vinblastine and bleomycin, along with methotrexate, a complete response has been achieved in a patient resistant to VAC. Alphafoetoproteins have a particular role here as tumour markers.

CONCLUSION

Ovarian cancer still presents in a very advanced form in more than 60% of cases. It is relatively responsive to a variety of treatments, but even in stages I and II the mortality rate is high. It would appear that adjuvant chemotherapy may prove helpful, and if such must be used, it appears that combination chemotherapy for six to 12 months only would be best, since the long-term use of alkylating agents is associated with a high incidence of acute leukaemia.

In stage III disease (less than 2 cm bulk), irradiation may have a role, but in bulky disease combination chemotherapy appears to be best. For stage III and stage IV disease, programmes of combination chemotherapy should be developed that are less toxic to the patient.

REFERENCES

1. Bagley, C. M., Young, R. C., Canellos, G. P., and DeVita, V. T. (1972): Treatment of ovarian carcinoma. *N. Engl. J. Med.*, 287:856–862.
2. Barker, G. H., and Wiltshawe, E. (1981): Cis-platinum and chlorambucil in advanced ovarian carcinoma. *Lancet*, 1:747–750.
3. Barr, W., Gowell, M. A. C., and Chatfield, W. R. (1970): The management of ovarian carcinoma: A review of 420 cases. *Scott. Med. J.*, 15:250–256.
4. Bush, R. S. (1979): *Malignancies of the Ovary, Uterus and Cervix*, pp. 65–66. Edward Arnold, London.
5. Decker, D. E., Malkasian, E. D., Jr., and Taylor, W. F. (1975): Prognostic importance of histological grading in ovarian carcinoma. *National Cancer Institute Monograph, Vol. 42, No. 9.*
6. DiSaia, P. J., Morrow, C. P., and Townsend, D. E. (1975): *Synopsis of Gynaecologic Oncology.* John Wiley & Sons, New York.
7. Fennelly, J. P. (1977): Treosulfan (dihydroxybusulfan) in the management of ovarian carcinoma. *Br. J. Obstet. Gynaecol.*, 84:300–303.
8. Hreshchyshyn, M. M. (1980): Role of adjuvant therapy in stage I ovarian carcinoma. *Am. J. Obstet. Gynecol.*, 138:139–145.
9. Kent, S. W., and McKay, D. E. (1960): Primary cancer of the ovary: An analysis of 349 cases. *Am. J. Obstet. Gynecol.*, 80:430–438.
10. Lokey, J., Baker, J. J., Price, N. A., and Winokur, S. H. (1981): Cisplatin, vinblastine, and bleomycin for endodermal sinus tumor of the ovary. *Ann. Intern. Med.*, 94:56–57.
11. Parker, L. M. (1980): Combination chemotherapy with adriamycin-cyclophossphamide for advanced ovarian carcinoma. *Cancer*, 46:669–674.
12. Pedersen-Bjergaard, J. (1980): Acute non-lymphocytic leukaemia in patients with ovarian carcinoma following long-term treatment with treosulfan. *Cancer*, 45:19–29.
13. Reimer, R. R., Hoover, R., Fraumeni, J. F., and Young, R. C. (1977): Acute leukemia after alkylating-agent therapy of ovarian cancer. *N. Engl. J. Med.*, 297:177–181.
14. Smith, J. P., and Rutledge, F. (1975): Advances in chemotherapy for gynecologic cancer. *Cancer*, 36:669–674.
15. Tobias, J. S., and Griffiths, C. T. (1976): Management of ovarian carcinoma (Parts I and II). *N. Engl. J. Med.*, 295:818–823.
16. Van Orden, D. E., McAllister, W. B., and Zerome, S. R. B. (1966): Ovarian carcinoma: The problems of staging and grading. *Am. J. Obstet. Gynecol.*, 94:195–202.
17. Wiltshawe, E. (1965): Chlorambucil in the treatment of primary adenocarcinoma of the ovary. *J. Obstet. Gynaecol. Br. Commonw.*, 72:586–594.
18. Young, R. C. (1978): Advanced ovarian carcinoma. *N. Engl. J. Med.*, 299:1261–1266.
19. Young, R. C., Hubbard, S. P., and DeVita, V. T. (1979): The chemotherapy of ovarian carcinoma. *Cancer Treat. Rev.*, 42:9–11.

Recent Clinical Developments in Gynecologic
Oncology, edited by C. Paul Morrow, et al.
Raven Press, New York © 1983.

Tumor Cell Sensitivity to Chemotherapeutic Agents Using a Modified Morley Procedure

*John A. Sykes, **Timothy J. O'Brien, and **C. Paul Morrow

*Southern California Cancer Center, Los Angeles, California, 90015; and
**Women's Hospital, University of Southern California Medical Center,
Los Angeles, California 90033

The observation that polyoma-transformed BHK 21/13 cells showed a 3 to 5 times higher transformation rate when plated in soft agar than when plated on glass indicated to Macpherson and Montagnier (6) that there was a highly significant correlation between transformation of cells by polyoma virus and their ability to form colonies in soft agar. Later, McAllister et al. (7) showed that cells of certain adenovirus-induced hamster tumors would form colonies in agar but that normal hamster cells would not. The colonies of cells showed histologic characteristics similar to those of the original tumors. McAllister and Reed (8) explored the soft agar technique to determine whether it could differentiate neoplastic from nonneoplastic tissues. They showed that cells from certain solid tumors of children formed colonies in agar but leukemic cells did not. Cells from normal human fetal tissues did not form colonies but cells from some diseased nonneoplastic hyperplastic lesions did. Courtenay et al. (1) grew cells from a human pancreatic carcinoma xenograft under reduced oxygen tension by the soft-agar technique using a replenishable liquid phase containing red blood cells. Later, Courtenay et al. (2) applied their soft-agar technique to cell suspensions from tumor tissue from 48 patients. Hamburger and Salmon (3) reported success in growing "human tumor stem cells" in a soft-agar medium. They made use of a feeder layer of agar-containing medium taken from adherent cultures of BALB/c mouse spleen cells. Using this technique, they were able to grow cells successfully from human bone marrow taken from patients with multiple myeloma, non-Hodgkin's lymphoma, chronic lymphocytic leukemia, oat-cell carcinoma of the lung, cells derived from lymph nodes of patients with melanoma, and ascitic cells from patients with adenocarcinoma of the ovary. Hamburger et al. (4) later reported on the direct cloning of human ovarian carcinoma cells in agar and made use of the technique to test the sensitivity of the cells to a chemotherapeutic agent, cis-platinum diamine dihydrochloride. They exposed single cell suspensions of the tumor cells to the action of the drug for 1 hr at 37°C before plating. By this method, they determined the sensitivity of the cells to the drug by comparing the number of colonies growing from drug-treated cell suspensions with the number of colonies obtained in the controls. Following the original observation of Macpherson and Montagnier (6), the soft-agar technique for clonogenic growth of tumor stem cells has become more widely used both for isolation of tumor cells (10,11,17) in culture and for assessment of the drug sensitivity of cells from different tumors (10,12,14). Salmon (13) has provided a good overview of the cloning of human tumor stem cells, and it appears to us that the soft-agar methodology holds great promise as a potent tool of the medical oncologist. As presently used for the determination of the sensitivity of human tumor stem cells to chemotherapeutic agents, the test is too subjective and unnecessarily laborious and cannot determine possible potentiations or antagonisms between different agents. This chapter details our preliminary studies of a simpler test using a modification of the Morley (9) procedure and the soft-agar technique, which is more objective and simple to perform and can determine potentiations and antagonisms between different agents.

MATERIALS AND METHODS

Culture Medium

The culture medium was minimum essential medium (Eagles) in powder form (Grand Island Biological Co., Grand Island, New York) reconstituted in triple distilled water and with the following additions designated as complete medium (CM). The additions were 15 mM Hepes, 10% heat-activated (56°C for 1 hr) fetal bovine serum, 200 ū/ml penicillin, 200 μg/ml streptomycin, 0.02 mg/ml bovine insulin (E. R. Squibb, Princeton, New Jersey), and 0.1 μg/ml human transferrin (Sigma Chemical Co., St. Louis, Missouri); sufficient 1 N NaOH solution was added to adjust the pH to 7.6 before sterilization by positive pressure filtration through a 0.01-μm Seitz filter pad. The CM was stored in 500-ml aliquots in screw-cap bottles kept at 5°C.

Trypsin-Versene Solution

The trypsin-Versene solution used to remove the cells from the glass T-30 culture flasks (Bellco Glass Co., Vineland, New Jersey) contained 0.25% trypsin 1:300 (Grand Island Biological Co.) and 0.01% disodium (ethylenedinitrilo-) tetracetate (Baker A. R., Phillipsburg, New Jersey) dissolved in Hanks balanced salt solution without calcium and magnesium salts in glass distilled water. 1 N NaOH solution was used to adjust the pH of the solution to 7.8 before sterilization by positive pressure filtration through a Seitz filter pad of 0.01-μm porosity. The sterile trypsin-Versene solution was stored at −22°C in 80-ml aliquots in screw-cap bottles.

Agar

In preliminary studies, Difco Bacto Agar, Difco Noble Agar, and Agarose were used. Although with the cell line used Bacto Agar was suitable, Noble Agar was selected because of its higher purity. Agarose overlayers were found to be too liquid at incubator temperature, permitting movement of colonies from convection currents. Stock agar solutions of 5 and 4% were prepared in 100-ml screw-cap bottles using 0.85% NaC1 solution as diluent. The bottles of agar were stored at room temperature.

Chemotherapeutic Agents

Suitable dilutions of various chemotherapeutic substances were prepared using triple-distilled water. Fresh dilutions of agents were prepared as dictated by the storage properties of the drug in solution listed by the manufacturer. The drug dilutions were applied to sterilized circles (6 mm diameter) of Whatman no. 2 ashless filter paper using a 10-μl "Oxford pipetter" with a tip sterilized by rinsing with 95% ethanol and washing with sterile-glass-distilled water. The discs with the different drug dilutions were placed in separate sterile 35-mm plastic dishes and incubated at 37°C for 1 to 2 hr before storage at 5°C. This procedure ensured that the drug dried into the filter paper. The concentrations of the drugs used in these studies were 1,000, 500, 100, 50, and 10 ng/disc Velban (vinblastine sulfate) and 500, 100, 50, and 10 ng/disc *cis*-platinum.

Cells

A well-established cell line, ME-180, derived in our laboratory from a human cervical carcinoma was used. The characteristics of ME-180 have been described previously (16). The cells were used at a concentration of 1×10^5 to 2×10^5 per ml. Cells were removed from the glass T-30 culture flasks when the culture was approaching confluence by exposure to trypsin-Versene solution for a period of 7 to 10 min at 37°C. The trypsin-Versene suspension of cells was diluted with CM to stop tryptic activity before pelleting by centrifugation at 5°C for 15 min at 1,000 $\times$ *g*. The supernatant fluid was removed, and the cells were resuspended in CM and counted using a hemocytometer. Because of the nature of the assay, residual clumps of cells did not affect the measurement of the zone of colony inhibition. The appropriate volume of cells in CM—1×10^5 per ml—was prepared and placed in a 39°C water bath to equilibrate before the addition of the required 1/10 volume of 4% agar solution cooled to 49°C just before plating.

Method

The required number of 60-mm plastic petri dishes was determined, and a base layer of CM containing 0.5% Noble Agar was pipetted into each dish, 3.0 ml per dish. The base layer was prepared from CM warmed to 39°C, to which was added sufficient melted 5% Noble Agar in 0.85% NaCl solution, which had been cooled to 49°C. The final agar concentration was 0.5%. After gelling of the base layer, the cell layer was prepared, and 2-ml aliquots were pipetted into each dish on top of the base layer. The cell layer was prepared by the addition to the cell suspension in CM of melted 4% Noble Agar in 0.85% NaCl solution cooled to 49°C. The final agar concentration in the cell suspension was 0.4%.

Following gelling of the cell layer, the dishes were labeled and the filter paper discs carrying the various drug concentrations placed in position in the center of the dish according to the labeling. The dishes were stacked on a simple carrier made to fit into a 1-gallon can. The cans, carriers, and the half-petri dish containing sterile distilled water to provide humidification were sterilized by autoclaving, and the polyethylene lids were sterilized by 75% ethanol. The cans were sealed adequately by the tight fit of the lids. The cultures were incubated at 37°C for 21 to 28 days. Following incubation, the dishes were removed and stained using an ethanol 0.02% solution of neutral red, about 2 ml per dish. The dishes were examined on an inverted microscope equipped with a 2.5× objective and 10× eyepieces. The radius of colony inhibition was easily measured, since the dishes had 2-mm squares engraved on the bottom (Falcon Plastics Div. B-D, Oxnard, California). When plain dishes were used, the zone was measured by placing a clear mm scale under the dish. A simpler method of measuring the zones is to use an opaque projector or comparator, which can provide a 4× to 10× image.

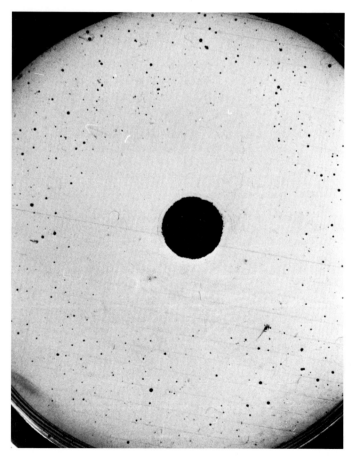

FIG. 1. 60-mm petri dish containing base layer of 3-ml CM with 0.5% Noble Agar overlaid with cell layer of 2-ml CM with 0.4% Noble Agar and 1 × 10⁵ ME-180 cells/ml. Incubated at 37°C in humidified atmosphere for 21 days. Radius of zone of colony inhibition was 12 mm with 100-ng Velban in disc. (×2.4)

Results

Figure 1, which is from a representative experiment, shows the effects of Velban on cells of ME-180. The cells were seeded in 2-ml aliquots per 60-mm dish of 0.4% agar containing CM with 1×10^5 cells per ml. The diameter of the filter paper discs was approximately 6 mm. The disc used for control plates was treated with 10-μl 0.85 NaCl solution instead of with one of the drugs being studied. When discs treated with 10-μl Velban at 100 ng/disc were placed on the cell overlay, a zone of inhibition of 12-mm radius was seen after 21 days incubation at 37°C in a humidified atmosphere (Fig. 1). Control dishes showed no inhibitory zone (Fig. 2) when incubated under the same conditions. When discs treated with 10-μl *cis*-platinum at 500 ng/disc were placed on the cell overlay and incubated in a similar

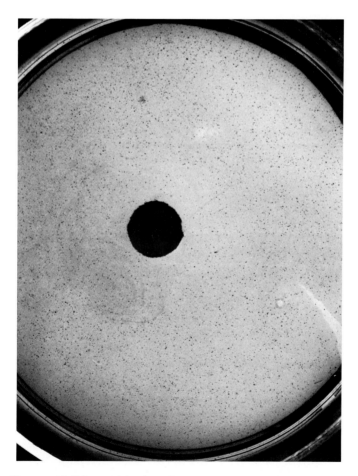

FIG. 2. 60-mm petri dish containing base layer of 3-ml CM with 0.5% Noble Agar overlaid with cell layer of 2-ml CM with 0.4% Noble Agar and 1×10^5 ME-180 cells/ml. Incubated at 37°C in humidified atmosphere for 21 days. No inhibition of colony formation was seen with 10-μl 0.85% NaCl solution in disc. (×2.4)

fashion, a zone of inhibition of 6-mm radius was observed (Fig. 3). The lower concentrations of both drugs used did not produce any objective colony inhibition, although routine screening of the dishes sometimes suggested that the colony size was smaller near the disc carrying the next lower concentration of the drug. Higher concentrations of both drugs generally resulted in no observable colonies on the dish, although on occasion plates with the next highest concentration did show a few scattered colonies near the periphery of the dish. The larger colony size seen in most dishes with zones of colony inhibition probably results from greater availability of nutrients rather than from a stimulatory effect of the drug. This observation is being studied.

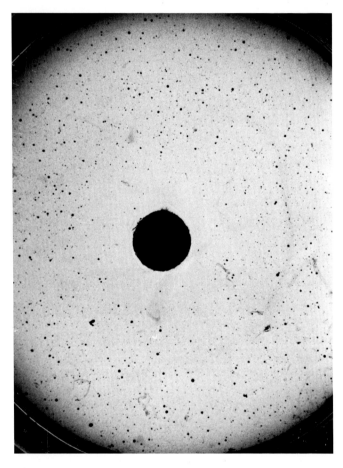

FIG. 3. 60-mm petri dish containing base layer of 3-ml CM with 0.5% Noble Agar overlaid with cell layer of 2-ml CM with 0.4% Noble Agar and 1 × 10⁵ ME-180 cells/ml. Incubated at 37°C in a humidified atmosphere for 21 days. The radius of the zone of colony inhibition was 6 mm, with 500 ng *cis*-platinum in disc. (×2.4)

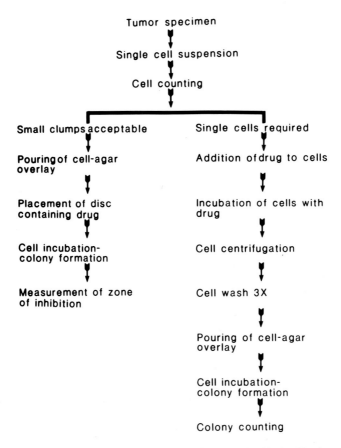

FIG. 4. Flow chart comparing the disc method (left channel) with the Hamburger-Salmon clonogenic assay procedure (right channel).

DISCUSSION

The original observation of Macpherson and Montagnier (6) that polyoma-virus-transformed BHK 21/13 cells had a higher transformation rate when plated in soft agar resulted in the use of this technique by McAllister et al. (7) to grow adenovirus-induced tumor cells from hamsters. Later, the growth of human tumor cells from children by McAllister and Reed (8) led to studies on growth of human tumor cells in this medium (3–5,10–12,15,17). These earlier studies on the use of a soft-agar medium for growth of tumor cells have been well summarized by Salmon (13). In the past 4 years, the use of this method for growing human tumor cells has progressed rapidly to the point where its use in screening human tumor cells for sensitivity to various drugs has become well accepted. The clonogenic assay for drug sensitivity of human tumor cells reported by Salmon (14), based on the earlier studies of Hamburger and Salmon (3), is being used in various centers as an aid toward better chemotherapy. The test, as currently used, appears to us to be too time consuming and rather subjective, depending as it does on colony counting. In an attempt to simplify drug-sensitivity testing of human tumor cells and to make the procedure more objective, we have used drug-carrying filter paper discs. The disc method gives results that are comparable to those obtained by the Salmon method but is faster and easier to carry out (Fig. 4). It gives more precise information on the drug sensitivity of the cells and permits construction of drug-sensitivity curves. The method also permits investigation of possible antagonisms and potentiations between different drugs and hormones.

These preliminary studies are being extended to the use of a wider spectrum of drugs. The development of sensitivity curves for these drugs against tumor cells should provide more precise data for the oncologist.

ACKNOWLEDGMENTS

This work was supported in part by contributions from the Albert Soiland Cancer Foundation, the California Hospital Medical Center, and by NIH Grant no. CA 20749.

REFERENCES

1. Courtenay, V. D., Smith, I. E., Peckham, M. J., and Steel, G. C. (1976): In vitro and in vivo radiosensitivity of human tumour cells obtained from a pancreatic carcinoma xenograft. *Nature*, 263:771–772.
2. Courtenay, V. D., Selby, P. J., Smith, I. E., Mills, J., and Peckham, M. J. (1978): Growth of human tumour cell colonies from biopsies using two soft agar techniques. *Br. J. Cancer*, 38:77–81.
3. Hamburger, A. W., and Salmon, S. E. (1977): Primary bioassay of human tumor stem cells. *Science*, 197:461–463.
4. Hamburger, A. W., Salmon, S. E., Kim, M. B., Trent, J. M., Soehnlen, B. J., Alberts, D. S., and Schmidt, H. J. (1978): Direct cloning of human ovarian carcinoma cells in agar. *Cancer Res.*, 38:3438–3444.
5. Hill, B. T., Whelan, R. D. M., Rupniak, H. T., and Rosholt, M. N. (1980): The value of an *in vitro* culture system for predicting drug sensitivities and their questionable clinical relevance. *Br. J. Cancer*, (Suppl. 4), 41:203.
6. Macpherson, I., and Montagnier, L. (1964): Agar suspension culture for the selective assay of cells transformed by polyoma virus. *Virology*, 23:291–294.
7. McAllister, R. M., Reed, G., and Huebner, R. J. (1967): Colonial growth in agar of cells derived from adenovirus-induced hamster tumors. *JNCI*, 39:43–53.
8. McAllister, R. M., and Reed, G. (1968): Colonial growth in agar of cells derived from neoplastic and non-neoplastic tissues of children. *Pediatr. Res.*, 2:356–360.
9. Morley, D. C. (1945): A simple method of testing the sensitivity of wound bacteria to penicillin and sulphathiazole by the use of impregnated blotting paper discs. *J. Path. Bact.*, 57:379–382.
10. Pavelic, Z. P., Slocum, H. K., Rustum, Y. M., Creaven, P. J., Karabousis, C., and Takita, H. (1980): Colony growth in soft agar of human melanoma, sarcoma and lung carcinoma cells disaggregated by mechanical and enzymatic methods. *Cancer Res.*, 40:2160–2164.
11. Pollard, E. B., Tio, F., Myers, J. W., Clark, G., Coltman Jr., C. A., and Van Hoff, D. D. (1981): Utilization of a human tumor cloning system to monitor marrow involvement with small cell carcinoma of the lung. *Cancer Res.*, 41:1015–1020.
12. Salmon, S. E. (1980): Applications of the human tumor stem cell assay to new drug evaluation and screening. *Prog. Clin. Biol. Res.*, 48:291–312.
13. Salmon, S. E. (1980): Cloning of human tumor stem cells: Background and overview. *Prog. Clin. Biol. Res.*, 48:3–13.

14. Salmon, S. E., Alberts, D. S., Durie, B. G. M., Meyskens, F. L., Jones, S. E., Soehnlen, B., Chen, H.-S. G., and Moon, T. (1980): Clinical correlations of drug sensitivity in the human tumor stem cell assay. *Recent Results Cancer Res.*, 74:300–305.
15. Salmon, S. E., Meyskens Jr., F. L., Alberts, D. S., Soehnlen, B., and Young, L. (1981): New drugs in ovarian cancer and malignant melanoma: In vitro phase II screening with the human tumor stem cell assay. *Cancer Treat. Rep.*, 65:1–12.
16. Sykes, J. A., Whitescarver, J., Jernstrom, P. J., Nolan, J. F., and Byatt, P. (1970): Some properties of a new epithelial cell line of human origin. *JNCI*, 45:107–122.
17. Van Hoff, D., Casper, J., Bradley, E., Trent, J. M., Modoch, A., Reichert, C., Makuch, R., and Altman, A. (1980): Direct cloning of human neuroblastoma cells in soft agar culture. *Cancer Res.*, 40:3591–3597.

Recent Clinical Developments in Gynecologic
Oncology, edited by C. Paul Morrow, et al.
Raven Press, New York © 1983.

Placental Proteins as Tumor Markers in Nontrophoblastic Malignancy

Timothy J. O'Brien and C. Paul Morrow

*University of Southern California School of Medicine, Division of Gynecologic Oncology,
Department of Obstetrics and Gynecology, Los Angeles, California 90033*

The usefulness of tumor markers originating from the placenta, more specifically from the syncytialtrophoblast, has become evident only in the past 25 years. A progression begun with the independent discovery and quantitation of human chorionic gonadotropin (hCG) by Hirose (23) in Japan and Ascheim and Zondek (1) in Germany has led to the characterization of many placental proteins. However, the real potential of trophoblastic tumor markers could not be appreciated until the introduction of the highly sensitive radioimmunoassay in 1958 by Berson and Yalow (4). Soon after, the hCG molecule was chemically characterized, providing the basis for the production of highly specific antibodies necessary for the hCG radioimmunoassay (3,11,48). The measurement of hCG in the serum and urine of patients with trophoblastic disease became the basis for diagnosis and therapy. As more highly specific and sensitive hCG assays became available, the threshold of sensitivity for serum hCG reached the value of approximately 1 mIU/ml. On the basis of the available standards and by comparing highly purified hCG on a mass basis, the value 1 mIU/ml translates into about 0.2 ng/ml using a conversion factor of 5 mIU to 1 ng. This threshold serum value for hCG is not detected in normal males or females and as such allows for almost complete discrimination between tumor-bearing patients and patients with no disease. The preceding data, of course, do not infer that the hCG molecule or any of the host of other trophoblastic tumor markers do not exist in the sera of normal men or nonpregnant women that are disease-free. On the contrary, there are significant data (7,10,50) indicating the presence of very low levels of hCG in both tissues and body fluids during normal metabolism and tissue turnover. These levels are below the sensitivity limits attainable under current assay conditions. However, it is inevitable that these limits will not remain for long and that the titration of abnormal levels of markers down to the normal basal range will soon be possible.

The existence of these marker proteins during normal tissue development and turnover and their amplification or apparent reappearance during carcinogenesis led

Pierce et al. (32) to describe neoplastic cells as caricatures of normal stem cells. This analogy provides a basis for understanding the increased presence of the so-called tumor-marker proteins during neoplastic growth. Neoplastic cells, owing to their increased numbers, produce larger quantities of normal stem-cell proteins compared to the quantities produced by the normal stem-cell population during differentiation and tissue renewal. On this basis, we may therefore anticipate that there are no unique tumor markers but only increased serum levels of normal differentiation proteins as a result of the accumulation of malignant cells. These conclusions suggest that protein markers may be useful eventually as monitors of normal tissue regeneration and as indicators of the accumulation of neoplastic cells. To develop a meaningful scheme for such monitoring, two major problems must be addressed: (a) which tumors produce which protein markers and (b) what the normal levels of such markers are in healthy individuals. This chapter will address the current status of the trophoblastic proteins hCG, placental lactogen (hPL), β_1-glycoprotein (SP$_1$), placental protein 5 (PP5), and the free subunits of hCG, that is, the alpha and beta subunits, as markers for gynecologic and nongynecologic tumors.

Several approaches to determining the presence or absence of such protein markers can be pursued. The most common approach is to evaluate the sera of tumor-bearing patients for the presence of increased protein-marker concentrations. This method provides some tenable avenues for the direct monitoring of tumor status. A second approach is possible when tumor tissue from patients is available, in which case the tumor can be directly analyzed for protein markers, and when present optimization of the secretion process can be attempted to make serum monitoring possible. A third approach, like the second, also utilizes tumor tissue, but instead of fresh tissue, formalin-fixed pathology specimens are screened for tumor markers with the highly sensitive immunoperoxidase system (45).

NORMAL SERUM LEVELS OF TROPHOBLASTIC PROTEINS

As a basis for the determination of abnormal concentrations of marker proteins, it is desirable to know the normal range of such proteins in both serum and tissue. For hCG, these values average 18–30 pg/ml in the sera of males and 101 pg/ml in the sera of females (Table 1). Tissue levels are relatively consistent from organ to organ, ranging from 12 to 26 ng/g tissue. The detection threshold of the most sensitive hCG assays is on the average 1 mIU/ml, which, when converted to grams, is 0.2 ng/ml (200 pg/ml). It therefore becomes obvious that the lower limits of the present assay for hCG detects concentrations of this molecule that are somewhat higher than the average normal circulating levels of the molecule but overlaps the upper normal range in females. The existence of SP$_1$ in the sera of disease-free nonpregnant individuals has also been documented (22,38,46). While normal tissue and serum concentrations have not been established, maximum serum levels of 4 ng/ml, 3.4 ng/ml, and 1.25 ng/ml have been detected in the sera of postmenopausal women, premenopausal women, and males, respectively (22).

TABLE 1. *Serum and tissue hCG levels in normal adults*

	No. cases	Average	Range
Serum			
Nonpregnant females	6	101 pg/ml	0–361 pg/ml
Males	10	30 pg/ml	0–103 pg/ml
Pool of normal men	13	18 pg/ml	—
Tissue			
Lung	5	18 ng/g tissue	10–26 ng/g tissue
Colon	5	16.5 ng/g tissue	12–21 ng/g tissue
Liver	5	18.3 ng/g tissue	15–21.5 ng/g tissue
Kidney	2	20.5 ng/g tissue	19–22 ng/g tissue

From Borkowski and Muguardt (7), Yoshimoto et al. (50), and Braunstein et al. (10).

hCG AS TUMOR MARKER

The excellence of hCG as a marker for gestational trophoblastic disease monitoring has been reviewed by Morrow et al. (30). As in the case of gestational trophoblastic disease, choriocarcinoma of the testes has been shown to produce hCG in 100% of cases (Table 2). Embryonal carcinoma and teratocarcinoma patients have hCG-positive sera in 50 to 60% of cases, while seminomas show a low incidence of hCG expression. The presence of low levels of hCG in marijuana users must be interpreted cautiously. One report of positive serum hCG in 2 postorchiectomy patients has been documented to be the result of heavy marijuana use (19). The hCG positivity disappeared 17 to 18 days after marijuana withdrawal.

A total of more than 1,200 cases of nontrophoblastic tumors evaluated by serum hCG assay is summarized in Table 3. Approximately 14% of cases were positive, with a higher incidence of positivity in ovarian, breast, skin, digestive-tract, and bronchial tumors. We have measured serum hCG in a series of patients with cervical, endometrial, and other gynecologic cancers. Elevated levels were found in 32 and 33% of cases, respectively, while only 1 of 6 ovarian, vulvar, and vaginal specimens

TABLE 2. *Frequency of elevated serum hCG levels in patients with testicular cancer*

Neoplasm	No. cases	% Positive
Seminoma	130	8
Embryonal carcinoma	145	60
Teratocarcinoma	56	57
Choriocarcinoma	5	100
Teratoma	16	25
Yolk-sac tumors	4	—
Total	356	39

From Javadpour (26,27).

TABLE 3. *Frequency of elevated serum hCG levels
in patients with nontrophoblastic malignancies*

Neoplasm	No. cases	% Positive
Ovarian	137	32
Bronchogenic	99	18
Digestive-tract	230	20
Melanoma	53	28
Breast	55	31
Leukemia	231	3
Multiple myeloma	93	9
Lymphoma	270	3
Sarcoma	46	13
Total	1,214	14

From Crowther et al. (14), Metz et al. (29), Gailani et al. (18), Samaan et al. (37), Goldstein et al. (20), Braunstein et al. (8), Stanhope et al. (41), and Stone et al. (42).

was positive (Table 4). It should be noted that the level of positivity in several serum samples was relatively high, reaching a value of 1,425 mIU/ml for the vulvar carcinoma case. These results are similar to those reported by other investigators (Table 5).

The presence of hCG in tumor extracts (cytosols) may be a more sensitive indicator of the potential usefulness of trophoblastic markers. In 75 cases of gynecologic tumors, we found 18% to have measurable amounts of hCG in the tumor extract (Table 6). Ovarian, endometrial, and cervical tumors were similar in that 17 to 21% were positive, while vulvar and vaginal tumors showed a lower level of positivity. The percentage of cytosols positive for hCG is lower than what we observed in the sera of patients with gynecologic malignancies, probably reflecting the relatively small number of cases.

TABLE 4. *Frequency of elevated serum hCG levels in patients with gynecologic malignancies[a]*

Neoplasm	No. cases	Positive No.	Positive %	Range (mIU/ml)
Malignant tumors				
Cervical	19	6	32	1–140
Endometrial	6	2	33	28–250
Ovarian, vulvar, vaginal	6	1	17	1,425[b]
Total	31	9	29	1–1,425
Benign tumors	23	1	4	2

[a]Authors' data.
[b]1,425 mIU/ml = metastic vulvar carcinoma.

TABLE 5. *hCG in serum of patients with gynecologic cancers*[a]

Neoplasm	No. cases	Positive No.	Positive %
Ovarian	286	100	35
Cervical, invasive	258	63	24
Cervical, *in situ*	66	5	8
Uterine, endometrial	167	26	16
Vulvar, vaginal	22	5	23

[a]Normal values varied from ≤ 0.5 mIU/ml to ≤ 10.0 mIU/ml.

From Sheth et al. (39), Crowther et al. (14), Samaan et al. (37), Braunstein et al. (8), Rosen (33), Rutanen and Seppala (36), Goldstein et al. (20), E. S. Donaldson et al. (15), C. R. Stanhope et al. (41), and M. Stone et al. (42).

ALPHA SUBUNIT OF GONADOTROPINS

Because the alpha subunit of hCG and other gonadotropins is synthesized independently of the beta subunit in amounts 6 to 10 times higher than the beta subunit, the alpha subunit has in and of itself been considered as a potential tumor marker. As in the case of the whole molecule of hCG, the free alpha subunit also is present in normal nontumor-bearing males and females (5) (Table 7). The highest circulating levels are in perimenopausal and postmenopausal women, while the lowest levels are in women on oral contraceptives and in men. Elevated serum levels of alpha subunit associated with nontrophoblastic tumors have been shown to be most common in melanoma and in thyroid and digestive-tract malignancies, ranging from 22 to 30% positivity (Table 8). The sera from patients with genital-tract tumors were found to be positive for the alpha subunit in 11% of cases. In malignant breast disease, the positivity rate for the free alpha subunit was shown to be significantly higher for tumor cytosols than for serum specimens, and, perhaps, higher for primary lesions than for metastatic lesions (Table 9). We found the

TABLE 6. *Cytosol hCG levels in gynecologic tumors*[a]

Neoplasm	No. cases	Positive No.	Positive %	Range (ng/mg protein)
Ovarian	15	3	20	0.2–15.5
Endometrial	30	5	17	3.25–24.0
Cervical	14	3	21	16.0–27.5
Vulvar, vaginal	16	2	7	17.0–160
Total	75	13	18	0.2–160

[a]Authors' data.

TABLE 7. *Normal circulating levels of free alpha subunit of hCG*

Group	Level (ng/ml)
Men	0.53
Premenopausal women	2.1
Perimenopausal women	3.52
Postmenopausal women	4.43
Women on oral contraceptives	<0.25

From Cove et al. (13), Rutanen (35), Shindelman et al. (40), and Dosogne-Guerin et al. (16).

cytosol levels of the alpha subunit in genital-tract tumors to be positive in 22% of cases (Table 10), but the maximum level detected was only 4.2 ng/mg protein. Of the malignancies evaluated for the alpha subunit using the immunoperoxidase staining technique, 23% of the primary breast tumors were shown to be positive, and in a small series, 100% of the bronchial and digestive-tract tumors (Table 11).

BETA SUBUNIT OF hCG

The free beta subunit of hCG has also been evaluated as a marker in nontrophoblastic tumors (Table 12). Cervical and thyroid cancers in the gathered data were shown to have the highest rates of positivity, amounting to 41 and 25%, respectively. In our genital-tract tumor cytosol series of 75 cases, 32% of endo-

TABLE 8. *Frequency of elevated serum hCG alpha-subunit levels in patients with nontrophoblastic tumors*

Neoplasm	No. cases	Positive No.	%
Malignant tumors			
Breast			
Primary stages I–IV	998	51	5
Metastatic	134	17	13
Genital-tract	146	16	11
Bronchogenic	51	6	12
Digestive-tract	37	8	22
Thyroid	12	3	25
Melanomas	20	6	30
Lymphomas and leukemias	29	1	—
Skin carcinomas	13	1	—
Pharynx and larynx	51	6	12
Miscellaneous	38	4	11
Total	1,529	96	6
Benign tumors	1,070	17	2

From Metz et al. (29), Rutanen (35), Shindelman et al. (40), Braunstein et al. (9), Dosogne-Guerin et al. (16), and Cove et al. (13).

TABLE 9. *Frequency of elevated hCG alpha-subunit levels in tumor cytosols of patients with breast cancer*

	No. cases	Positive	
		No.	%
Primary stages I–IV	181	62	34
Metastatic	37	10	28

From Cove et al. (13), Shindelman et al. (40), and Cove et al. (12).

metrial carcinomas were found to be positive for the free beta subunit of hCG, although the level of positivity was not much higher than the sensitivity of the assay (Table 13).

PREGNANCY-SPECIFIC β_1-GLYCOPROTEIN (SP$_1$)

A relatively new addition to the tumor marker list is SP$_1$. It has been described by several synonyms (Table 14), but the most commonly used name is pregnancy-

TABLE 10. *Frequency of elevated hCG alpha-subunit cytosol levels in gynecologic cancers[a]*

Neoplasm	No. cases	Positive		Range (ng/mg protein)
		No.	%	
Ovarian	15	4	27	0.03–0.8
Endometrial	30	8	27	0.03–4.2
Cervical	14	2	14	0.09–1.68
Vulvar, vaginal	16	2	13	0.10–1.03
Total	75	16	22	0.03–4.2

[a]Authors' data.

TABLE 11. *Frequency of hCG alpha subunit in nontrophoblastic tumors by immunoperoxidase method*

Neoplasm	No. cases	Positive	
		No.	%
Breast, primary	58	13	23
Bronchogenic	5	5	100[a]
Digestive-tract	17	17	100[a]

[a]Positive also for LH-releasing hormone.
From Wahlstrom and Seppala (49) and Cove et al. (12).

TABLE 12. *Frequency of elevated serum hCG beta-subunit levels in patients with nontrophoblastic tumors*

	No. cases	Positive	
Neoplasm		No.	%
Malignant tumors			
Breast	220	25	10
Cervical	32	13	41
Bronchial	50	6	12
Digestive-tract	37	7	19
Genital-tract	45	7	16
Thyroid	12	3	25
Melanomas	20	3	15
Lymphomas and leukemias	29	3	10
Skin carcinomas	13	2	15
Pharynx and larynx	51	3	6
Miscellaneous	38	7	18
Total	547	79	14
Benign tumors	99	16	16

From Sheth et al. (39), Cove et al. (13), and Dosogne-Guerin et al. (16).

specific β_1-glycoprotein. This trophoblastic protein has already been found to be a useful adjuvant serum marker in trophoblastic disease monitoring (31). It has also been evaluated for use as a marker in testicular cancer (Table 15). In general, the

TABLE 13. *Cytosol hCG beta-subunit levels in gynecologic malignancies[a]*

Neoplasm	No. cases	Positive		Range (ng/mg protein)
		No.	%	
Ovarian	15	3	20	0.2–0.95
Endometrial	30	8	32	0.2–2.0
Cervical	14	1	7	3.5
Vulvar, vaginal	16	2	7	0.8–7.31
Total	75	14	19	0.2–7.31

[a]Authors' data.

TABLE 14. *Synonyms for SP$_1$*

Name	Ref.
Beta globulin	43
Trophoblastic specific β_1-glycoprotein (TBG)	44
Schwangerschafts-Spezifische Protein eins (SP$_1$)	6
Pregnancy-associated plasma protein (PAPP-C)	28
Pregnancy-specific β_1-glycoprotein (SP$_1$)	46

TABLE 15. *Serum SP₁ in testicular cancer patients*

	No. cases	Positive	
Neoplasm		No.	%
Seminoma	32	0	0
Choriocarcinoma	6	3	50
Teratoma and teratocarcinomas	18	6	33
Embryonal carcinoma	50	5	10
Total	106	14	13

From Rosen et al. (34) and Grudzinskas et al. (21).

pattern of SP_1 serum levels in testicular cancer patients follows that of hCG, with perhaps a lowered positivity rate owing to the reduced sensitivity of the present assay for SP_1 (47). As a serum marker for nontrophoblastic tumors, SP_1 has been found to have the highest positivity rate in liver and colorectal cancers (Table 16). In ovarian cancer, a positivity rate of 13% was observed. When SP_1 was evaluated in tissue sections of a variety of tumors using the immunoperoxidase screening method, a high rate of positivity was detected in tumors of the colon, breast, digestive tract, and lung (Table 17).

hPL

The protein hPL has been known for several years but until recently has not attracted much attention as a potential tumor marker. In a series of 147 patients with ovarian or cervical tumors, serum hPL was found to have a high positivity rating (Table 18). Although there exists a large discrepancy between the rate of

TABLE 16. *Serum SP₁ in nontrophoblastic tumors*

	No. cases	Positive	
Neoplasm		No.	%
Breast	91	8	9
Digestive-tract	43	1	—
Lung	40	2	—
Melanoma	41	1	—
Sarcoma	4	0	—
Liver	14	3	21
Colon-rectum	39	11	28
Ovarian	60	8	13
Uterine	6	1	—
Miscellaneous	49	1	—
Total	387	36	9

From Grudzinskas et al. (21), Engvall and Yonemoto (17), Bagshawe et al. (2), Crowther et al. (14), Searle et al. (38), and Tatarinov and Sokolov (44).

TABLE 17. *Frequency of SP₁ presence in nontrophoblastic tumors by immunoperoxidase method*

Neoplasm	No. cases	Positive	
		No.	%
Breast	69	48	70
Gastric	12	8	66
Colon	4	4	100
Lung	3	2	66
Ovarian	7	0	0
Endometrial	3	0	0
Total	98	62	63

From Inaba et al. (25) and Horne et al. (24).

elevated serum values for hPL in patients with ovarian tumors, 22% of one series of 37 cases (14) and 72% of another series of 65 cases (37), hPL obviously has potential as a tumor marker and deserves further study.

PP5

Placental protein 5, a recent addition to the list of placental proteins secreted during pregnancy, has been shown to have a high positivity rate by the immuno-peroxidase method in breast, testicular, and endometrial tumors (Table 19).

DISCUSSION

The unique success of hCG as a tumor marker for trophoblastic tumors has served both as a stimulus to search for markers produced by nontrophoblastic tumors and as a standard by which the usefulness of all such marker substances can be judged. In our study we focused attention on glycoproteins that, like hCG, are normal

TABLE 18. *Serum hPL in nontrophoblastic gynecologic cancer patients*

Neoplasm	No. cases	Positive	
		No.	%
Ovarian	37	8	22
Cervical	45	27	60
Ovarian	65	47	72
Total	147	82	56

From Crowther et al. (14), Sheth et al. (39), and Samaan et al. (37).

TABLE 19. *Frequency of PP5
identification in nontrophoblastic tumors
by immunoperoxidase method*

Neoplasm	No. cases	Positive	
		No.	%
Breast	69	53	77
Testicular	24	18	75
Colon	4	1	—
Stomach	12	5	42
Lung	3	1	—
Ovarian	7	2	29
Endometrial	3	2	66
Total	72	41	57

From Inaba et al. (25) and Horne et al. (24).

secretory products of placental tissue. The fact that placental proteins are mainfested in nontrophoblastic tumors has only recently come to general attention. It is also apparent that the level of expression of these proteins in nontrophoblastic tumors is greatly diminished compared to that in trophoblastic disease. For this reason alone, we cannot expect the existing detection systems to be sensitive enough to fully appreciate the subtle changes in protein concentration that would occur during the early growth of any malignancy. For example, the hCG values in normal males and females are presently well out of range of the standard hCG assay, namely, a maximum sensitivity of 200 pg/ml for the assay and an average of 18 to 30 pg/ml in normal males and 100 pg/ml in normal females. The present assay system therefore may not detect many hCG-positive tumors. While reduced expression of placental protein in nontrophoblastic tumors is a problem, an increased sensitivity in the assay's system may overcome much of this difficulty.

Direct analysis of tumor extracts could be a very useful means of identifying potential serum tumor markers. Because placental proteins manifested by the tumor are more concentrated in malignant tissue than in the serum, the measurement of protein markers in tumor tissue provides a reasonable indication of the false-negative rate caused by inherent insensitivity of the current serum assay methodology. The recent addition of the highly sensitive immunoperoxidase-staining procedure of tissue sections embedded in Formalin (formaldehyde solution) (45) adds further possibilities to the screening of tumor tissue for marker proteins. This procedure would allow testing for many antigens with a minimum amount of tumor tissue available even on a retrospective basis. At the present time, quantitation of antigen concentration in the immunoperoxidase system is not easily attainable and therefore some limitations still exist with this method.

The frequency with which measurable levels of placental proteins are present in the serum or tumor tissue from patients with nontrophoblastic malignancies is often in the 10 to 50% range and can be even higher when immunoperoxidase testing is utilized. If the quantity of marker protein secreted were higher, there is no question that these substances would be extremely valuable markers for tumor activity and treatment response. There is good reason to believe that the assay sensitivity can be substantially improved, but the benefits of this approach apparently will be limited by naturally occurring low levels of these proteins in healthy nonpregnant individuals. This is certainly well documented for hCG. The source of the placental proteins in healthy human subjects is postulated to be the normal stem cells of replicating tissues, which like the stem cells of malignant tumors are very primitive or undifferentiated, a property they have in common with normal trophoblastic tissue.

Although the reason is not clear, there is a general tendency for the placental proteins to be more often associated with nontrophoblastic tumors of the female genital tract than with other malignancies. It may then be expected that the measurement of one or more of these markers may have become accepted as an integral part of gynecologic cancer surveillance. However, this does not appear to be true even for hCG, which has received the most attention. This unspoken judgment does not seem to be entirely warranted, certainly not on the basis of our limited experience. Among 31 patients with gynecologic malignancies (Table 4), 3 had serum hCG values between 140 and 1,400 mIU/ml, levels entirely consistent with surveillance of tumor response to treatment and surveillance after treatment. Evaluation of the other placental proteins—hPL, SP_1, and PP5—is just beginning.

In conclusion, early indications that placental proteins are synthesized by some nontrophoblastic tumor cells are well founded. The level of expression of such proteins is significantly lower than in trophoblastic cells and therefore necessitates increased sensitivity in the assay systems for full appreciation of their presence. In contrast to the syncytiotrophoblast, which synthesizes all of the placental proteins known to be secreted, nontrophoblastic tumors usually manifest none or only one of these proteins. The task of selecting which patients are suitable for monitoring by which protein assay is necessary. It is apparent that placental proteins not only are manifested in normal tissues but can reach relatively high levels in nonmalignant disorders. The documentation of such expression is just beginning, and as such, consideration must be given to the possibility that marker protein positivity may not be related to malignancy in individual cases. Finally, it is clear that none of the placental proteins has been fully assessed for its potential as a marker for gynecologic nontrophoblastic malignancy.

REFERENCES

1. Ascheim, S., and Zondek, B. (1928): Die schwangerschafts Diagnose aus dem Harn durch Machieveis des hypophysenvorder Lappen-Hormons. Klin. Wochenschr., 7:1404–1411.
2. Bagshawe, K. D., Lequin, R. M., Sizaret, P. H., and Tatarinov, Y. S. (1978): Pregnancy β_1 glycoprotein and chorionic gonadotropin in the serum of patients with trophoblastic and nontrophoblastic tumors. Eur. J. Cancer., 14:1331–1335.
3. Bahl, O. P., Carlsen, R. B., Bellisaris, R., and Swaminathan, K. (1972): Human chorionic gonadotropin: Amino-acid sequence of alpha and beta subunits. Biochem. Biophys. Res. Commun., 48:416–422.
4. Berson, S. A., and Yalow, R. S. (1958): Isotopic tracers in the study of diabetes. Adv. Biol. Med. Phys., 6:350–354.

5. Blackman, M. R., Weintraub, B. D., Kourides, I. A., Solano, J. T., Santer, T., and Rosen, S. W. (1981): Discordant elevation of the common α-subunit of the glycoprotein hormones compared to β-subunits in serum of uremic patients. *J. Clin. Endocrinol. Metab.*, 53:39–48.

6. Bohn, H. (1971): Nachweis und Charakterisierung von Schwangschafts-Protein in der manschlichen Placenta, Sowie ihre quantitative immunologische Bestimmung im serum schwangerer Frauen. *Arch. Gynaek.*, 210:440–457.

7. Borkowski, A., and Muguardt, C. (1979): Human chorionic gonadotropin in the plasma of normal, non-pregnant subjects. *N. Engl. J. Med.*, 301:298–302.

8. Braunstein, G. D., Vaitukaitis, J. L., Carbone, P. P., and Ross, G. T. (1973): Ectopic production of human chorionic gonadotrophin by neoplasms. *Ann. Intern. Med.*, 78:39–45.

9. Braunstein, G. D., Forsythe, A. B., Rasor, J. L., Van Scoy Mosher, M. B., Thompson, R. W., and Wade, M. E. (1979): Serum glycoprotein hormone alpha subunit levels in patients with cancer. *Cancer*, 44:1644–1651.

10. Braunstein, G. D., Kandar, V., Rasor, J., Swaminathan, M., and Wade, M. E. (1979): Widespread distribution of a chorionic gonadotropin-like substance in normal human tissues. *J. Clin. Endocrinol. Metab.*, 49:917–925.

11. Canfield, R. E., Morgan, F. J., Kammerman, S., Bell, J. J., and Agosto, G. M. (1971): Studies of human chorionic gonadotropin. *Recent. Prog. Horm. Res.*, 27:121–164.

12. Cove, D. H., Smith, S. C. H., Walker, R., and Howell, A. (1979): The synthesis of the glycoprotein hormone a subunit by human breast carcinomas. *Eur. J. Cancer*, 15:693–702.

13. Cove, D. H., Woods, K. L., Smith, S. C. H., Burnett, D., Leonard, J., Grieve, R. J., and Howell, A. (1979): Tumor markers in breast cancer. *Br. J. Cancer*, 40:710–718.

14. Crowther, M. E., Grudzinskas, J. G., Poulton, T. A., and Gordon, Y. B. (1979): Trophoblastic proteins in ovarian carcinoma. *Obstet. Gynecol.*, 53:59–61.

15. Donaldson, E. S., Van Nagell, J. R., Pursell, S., Gay, E. C., Meeker, W. R., Kashmiri, R., and Van de Voorde, J. (1980): Multiple biochemical markers in patients with gynecologic malignancies. *Cancer*, 45:948–953.

16. Dosogne-Guérin, M., Stolarczyk, A., and Borkowski, A. (1978): Prospective study of the alpha and beta subunits of human chorionic gonadotrophin in the blood of patients with various benign and malignant conditions. *Eur. J. Cancer*, 14:525–532.

17. Engvall, E., and Yonemoto, R. H. (1979): Is SP_1 (pregnancy specific β_1 glycoprotein) elevated in cancer patients? *Int. J. Cancer*, 23:759–761.

18. Gailani, S., Ming, C. T., Nussbaum, A., Ostrander, M., and Christoff, N. (1976): Human chorionic gonadotrophins (hCG) in non-trophoblastic neoplasms: Assessment of abnormalities of hCG and CEA in bronchogenic and digestive neoplasms. *Cancer*, 38:1684–1686.

19. Garnick, M. B. (1980): Spurious rise in human chorionic gonadotropin induced by marijuana in patients with testicular cancer. *N. Engl. J. Med.*, 303:1177.

20. Goldstein, D. P., Kosasa, T. S., and Skarin, A. T. (1974): The clinical application of a specific radioimmunoassay for human chorionic gonadotropin in trophoblastic and non-trophoblastic tumors. *Surg. Gynecol. Obstet.*, 138:747–751.

21. Grudzinskas, J. G., Coombes, R. C., Ratcliffe, J. G., Gordon, Y. B., Powles, T. J., Neville, A. M., and Chard, T. (1980): Circulating levels of pregnancy-specific B_1 glycoprotein in patients with testicular bronchogenic and breast carcinomas. *Cancer*, 45:102–103.

22. Haase, H. R. (1978): Radioimmunoassay of pregnancy specific β_1-glycoprotein. *M.S. Thesis*, University of Sydney.

23. Hirose, T. (1920): Exogenous stimulation of corpus luteum formation in the rabbit; Influence of extracts of human placenta, decidua, fetus and hydatidiform mole and bovine corpus luteum on the rabbit gonad. *J. Jpn. Gynecol. Soc.*, 16:1055.

24. Horne, C. H. W., Reid, I. N., and Milne, G. D. (1976): Prognostic significance of inappropriate production of pregnancy proteins by breast cancers. *Lancet*, 2:279–282.

25. Inaba, N., Renk, T., Wurster, K., Rapp, W., and Bohn, H. (1980): Ectopic synthesis of pregnancy specific β_1-glycoprotein (SP₁) and placental specific tissue proteins (PP₅, PP₁₀, PP₁₁, PP₁₂) in non-trophoblastic malignant tumors. Possible markers in oncology. *Klin Wochenschr.*, 58:789–791.

26. Javadpour, N. (1979): Applications of biologic tumor markers in testicular cancer. *Cancer Treat. Rep.*, 63:1643–1647.

27. Javadpour, N. (1980): The role of biologic tumor markers in testicular cancer. *Cancer*, 45:1755–1761.

28. Lin, T. M., Halbert, S. P., and Kiefer, D. (1973): Pregnancy-associated serum antigens in the rat and mouse. *Proc. Soc. Exp. Biol. Med.*, 145:62–66.

29. Metz, S., Weintraub, B., Singer, J., and Robertson, R. P. (1978): Ectopic secretion of chorionic gonadotropin by a lung carcinoma. *Am. J. Med.*, 65:325–333.
30. Morrow, C. P., O'Brien, T. J., and Schlaerth, J. (1981): Is human chorionic gonadotropin the ideal tumor marker? In: *Gynecologic Oncology, Controversies in Cancer Treatment*, edited by S. C. Ballon, pp. 376–394. G. K. Hall, Boston.
31. O'Brien, T. J., Engvall, E. Schlaerth, J., and Morrow, C. P. (1980): Trophoblastic disease monitoring: Evaluation of pregnancy-specific β_1-glycoprotein. *Am. J. Obstet. Gynecol.*, 138:313–320.
32. Pierce, G. B., Shikes, R., and Fink, L. M. (1978): Tumours as caricatures of tissue renewal. In: *Cancer: A Problem of Developmental Biology*, pp. 27–47. Prentice-Hall, Englewood Cliffs, New Jersey.
33. Rosen, S. W. (1975): Placental proteins and their subunits as tumor markers. *Ann. Intern. Med.*, 82:71–83.
34. Rosen, S. W., Javadpour, N., Calvert, I., and Kaminska, J. (1979): Increased pregnancy-specific Beta1-glycoprotein in certain non-seminomatous germ cell tumors. *JNCI*, 62:1439–1441.
35. Rutanen, E. M. (1978): The circulating alpha subunit of human chorionic gonadotrophin in gynaecologic tumours. *Int. J. Cancer*, 22:413–421.
36. Rutanen, E. M., and Seppala, M. (1978): The hCG-subunit radioimmunoassay in non-trophoblastic gynecologic tumors. *Cancer*, 41:692–696.
37. Samaan, N., Smith, J. P., Rutledge, F. N., and Schultz, P. N. (1976): The significance of measurement of human placental lactogen, human chorionic gonadotropin, and carcinoembryonic antigen in patients with ovarian carcinoma. *Am. J. Obstet. Gynecol.*, 126:186–189.
38. Searle, F., Leake, B. A., Bagshawe, K. K., and Dent, J. (1978): Serum SP₁-pregnancy-specific-β-glycoprotein in choriocarcinoma and other neoplastic disease. *Lancet*, 1:579–581.
39. Sheth, N., Adil, M., Nadkarni, J., Rajpal, R. M., and Sheth, A. R. (1981): Inappropriate secretion of human placental lactogen and β-subunit of human chorionic gonadotropin by cancer of the uterine cervix. *Gynecol. Oncol.*, 11:321–329.
40. Shindelman, J. E., Ortmeyer, A. E., Wada, H. G., Stockdale, F., and Sussman, H. H. (1980): Distribution and characterization of alpha hCG in the serum and tumor cytosol of patients with breast cancer. *Int. J. Cancer*, 25:599–604.
41. Stanhope, C. R., Smith, J. P., Britton, J. C., and Crosby, P. K. (1979): Serial determination of marker substances in ovarian cancer. *Gynecol. Oncol.*, 8:284–287.
42. Stone, M., Bagshawe, K. D., Kardana, A., and Searle, F. B. (1977): Human chorionic gonadotropin and carcino-embryonic antigen in the management of ovarian carcinoma. *Br. J. Obstet. Gynaecol.*, 84:375–379.
43. Tatarinov, Y. S., and Masyukevich, V. M. (1970): Immunological identification of a new beta 1-globulin in the blood serum of pregnant women. *Biull. Eksp. Biol. Med.*, 69:66–68.
44. Tatarinov, Y. S., and Sokolov, A. J. (1977): Development of a radioimmunoassay for pregnancy-specific beta 1-globulin and its measurement in serum of patients with trophoblastic and non-trophoblastic tumours. *Int. J. Cancer*, 19:161–166.
45. Taylor, C. R. (1978): Immunoperoxidase techniques. *Arch. Pathol. Lab. Med.*, 102:113–121.
46. Towler, C. M., Jandial, V., Horne, C. H. W., and Bohn, H. (1976): A serial study of pregnancy proteins in primigravida. *Br. J. Obstet. Gynaecol.*, 83:368–374.
47. Towler, C. M., Horne, C. H. W., Jandial, V., and Chesworth, J. M. (1977): A simple and sensitive radioimmunoassay for pregnancy-specific β_1-glycoprotein. *Br. J. Obstet. Gynaecol.*, 84:580–584.
48. Vaitukaitis, J. L., Braunstein, G. D., and Ross, G. T. (1972): A radioimmunoassay which specifically measures human chorionic gonadotropin in the presence of luteinizing hormone. *Am. J. Obstet. Gynecol.*, 113:751–758.
49. Wahlstrom, T., and Seppala, M. (1981): Immunological evidence for the occurrence of luteinizing hormone-releasing factor and the α-subunit of glycoprotein hormones in carcinoid tumors. *J. Clin. Endocrinol. Metab.*, 53:209–212.
50. Yoshimoto, Y., Wolfsen, A. R., Hirose, F., and Odell, W. D. (1979): Human chorionic gonadotropin-like material: Presence in normal human tissues. *Am. J. Obstet. Gynecol.*, 134:729–733.

Recent Clinical Developments in Gynecologic Oncology, edited by C. Paul Morrow, et al. Raven Press, New York © 1983.

Laparoscopy in Gynecologic Oncology

Conley G. Lacey

Department of Obstetrics and Gynecology, University of California, San Francisco, San Francisco, California 94117

Laparoscopy for the evaluation of intra-abdominal disorders has been employed since the turn of the century, particularly in Europe. In 1937, Ruddock (9), an internist from the University of Southern California, reported his experience with laparoscopy on 500 patients, many of whom had intra-abdominal cancers. Despite his enthusiasm and early success, the technique was not used for the evaluation of gynecologic cancers to any significant degree until the early 1970s, when reports appeared in the literature suggesting a role for laparoscopy as a second-look procedure in ovarian cancer. Over the past decade, somewhat less than 1,000 laparoscopically evaluated gynecologic cancer patients have been reported. Some authors have recommended it for pretreatment evaluation or restaging of ovarian cancer patients referred for chemotherapy following exploration, while others have used it as a surveillance procedure to follow regression or progression of peritoneal metastases during chemotherapy. Today, the most popular indication for laparoscopy in gynecologic oncology is the second-look procedure to confirm the presence or absence of disease following chemotherapy. Theoretically, this indication has the greatest potential, but somewhat unexpectedly laparoscopy has met with varying success when used for this purpose.

Despite a growing interest in laparoscopy among gynecologic oncologists, there are still several other unexplored areas that need study. Cervical cancer and endometrial cancer, for example, are known to follow a spread pattern similar to epithelial ovarian carcinoma when they invade the peritoneal cavity, yet there exists no adequate study using laparoscopy to evaluate this mode of dissemination in advanced stages of such cancers.

This chapter presents the author's experience using laparoscopy to evaluate patients with a variety of suspected or proven gynecologic neoplasms and compares them with similar patients reported in the literature.

INDICATIONS, PATIENT SELECTION, AND TECHNIQUE

Initially, patients were selected for laparoscopy if they had serious medical problems or were thought to have such advanced disease that laparotomy may prove unnecessary or hazardous. As personal experience with the procedure in cancer patients has grown and reports of others have appeared, distinct areas of study have evolved. The indications for laparoscopy in this group fall into several broad categories: (a) staging laparoscopy, used in patients without previous treatment or intra-abdominal evaluation, (b) surveillance laparoscopy, used in patients with suspected recurrence or to follow the progression or regression of disease during adjuvant therapy or to restage patients referred for chemotherapy, (c) diagnostic laparoscopy, used in patients with pelvic masses suspected of being malignant, and (d) second-look laparoscopy, used in patients with no clinical evidence of disease following completion of adjuvant chemotherapy.

Since 1971, 92 patients with a wide range of suspected or proven pelvic neoplasms have been evaluated: 50 patients for ovarian cancer, 31 for cervical cancer, and 11 for other suspected gynecologic or visceral neoplasms. In general, they were older, at relatively high operative risk by virtue of their age, obesity, medical infirmity, previous abdominal surgery, or previous pelvic or abdominal radiation therapy (Table 1). Forty-seven patients (51%) had at least 1 previous laparotomy, and 28 (30%) had previous pelvic radiation therapy, including 3 that received intraperitoneal radioactive chromic phosphate (32^P). Patients with extensive abdominal scarring, a history of peritonitis, or extensive bowel surgery were considered unsuitable for laparoscopy, as were patients with bowel fistulae. Previous laparotomies, abdominal radiation, or obesity in themselves did not preclude the procedure.

General anesthesia was preferred and is considered essential in most instances, since it allows greater distention of the abdomen by the pneumoperitoneum than does local anesthesia; general anesthesia also facilitates manipulation of the viscera by ancillary instruments. Moreover, and perhaps most importantly, with general anesthesia the operating table can be tilted considerably to the head-up or head-down position, causing the viscera to fall away from the diaphragm or out of the pelvis as the case may be. Support stirrups are used to keep the legs spread apart and horizontal, thereby allowing the laparoscopist optimum working space. When the end of the table is lowered, the surgeon can stand between the patient's legs to view the epigastrium and diaphragms, an integral part of the evaluation.

A standard laparoscopic technique using a subumbilical incision was utilized in all but 3 patients. When a midline scar was present, the Verres needle was directed laterally to it but medial to the true pelvic brim to avoid injuring the iliac vessels. When the midline approach was considered perilous because of extensive scarring, a left upper quadrant incision located near the costal margin and the rectus border was used.

TABLE 1. *Age, height, and weight*
of group in study

	Mean	Range
Age	50	16–89
Weight (lb.)	140	84–230
Height (in.)	63	59–70

The intraperitoneal position of the needle was always confirmed by the audible sign (2), pressure gauge changes, and the rapid disappearance of liver dullness. In the early years of the study, if the position of the needle was in doubt, the procedure was abandoned rather than risk injury, but now under these circumstances, laparoscopy is performed through a very small incision (open laparoscopy).

COMPLICATIONS

One episode of peritonitis following fundal biopsy of an infected cervical car cinoma was the only major complication of this series. When compared to the reported incidence of serious complications (Table 2), the patients have fared well (5–9). Similarly, the 10% incidence of unsuccessful or inadequate procedures is similar to that reported in the literature (Table 3).

Because of the frequent history of prior surgery or radiation therapy in patients undergoing laparoscopy for the evaluation of gynecologic cancer, bowel injury, not

TABLE 2. *Reported incidence of serious complications, collected series*

Year	Ref.	Procedures	Complications	%
1981	1[a]	119	8	7
1981	5[a,b]	159	6	4
1980	7	110	3	3
1980	6	22	0	0
1979	4	123	1	1
1977	10	24	0	0
1976	11	95	0	0
1982	This chapter	92	1	1
	Total	744	19	2.5

[a]If these two series are excluded, the incidence is 5/466 (1%).
[b]Pneumomediastinum included as a major complication.

TABLE 3. *Reported incidence of unsuccessful or inadequate procedures*

Year	Ref.	Procedures	Unsuccessful	%
1981	1	119	16	13
1981	5[a]	159	9	6
1980	7	110	14	3
1980	6	22	0	0
1979	4	123	25	21
1977	10	24	5	21
1982	This chapter	92	9	10
	Total	649	78	12

[a]Many more patients with inadequate pelvic visualization.

TABLE 4. *Reported serious complications*

Complication	No. cases	Ref.
Bowel perforation, repaired	11	(1)
		(7)
		(4)
Hemorrhage	2	(1)
		(5)
Hypotension	2	(5)
Pneumothorax	2	(5)
		(10)
Pneumomediastinum	1	(5)
Peritonitis	1	(3)

unexpectedly, is the most commonly reported serious complication (Table 4). However, as investigators have become more familiar with the technique in high-risk patients and have introduced precautionary measures, such as open laparoscopy and antecedent needle laparoscopy, the occurrence of bowel perforation has diminished. Nevertheless, in most instances these measures should not be necessary if one adheres to the technical measures described above.

OVARIAN CANCER

Fifty patients in this series were laparoscoped for the evaluation of suspected or known ovarian cancer. In 19 cases, the procedure was performed to diagnose the etiology of a pelvic mass simulating ovarian cancer in patients who, for medical or other reasons, were not good laparotomy candidates. Three of the 19 patients were found to have resectable ovarian cancer, and another 5 were found to have benign ovarian neoplasms requiring resection. Two patients had unresectable ovarian carcinomatosis, and 1 patient had unresectable widespread visceral metastases from an unknown primary. Eight patients had benign conditions, such as broad ligament fibroids or diverticulosis, that did not require surgery. Therefore, 11 of the 19 patients (58%) had benign or unresectable lesions that did not require further surgery, while 8 of the 19 (42%) required laparotomy for resection.

Twenty-one ovarian cancer patients without clinical evidence of disease following adjuvant chemotherapy underwent laparoscopy as a second-look procedure to determine future treatment (Table 5). Only one of 12 stage I and stage II patients had positive findings at laparoscopy, but these patients were at low risk for recurrence because of low-stage or well-differentiated tumors at the time of original surgery. Of the 11 stage I and stage II patients who had a negative laparoscopy, 5 underwent a sequential laparotomy, which proved to be negative in each case. The remaining 6 patients were considered of such low risk for recurrence that a full second-look laparotomy was not performed. Nine stage III and stage IV patients underwent second-look laparoscopy, and 3 had unresectable disease. Of the 6 stage III and stage IV patients that had a negative laparoscopy, 4 underwent a sequential laparotomy, and recurrent disease was identified in 3. At laparoscopy, 2 of the 3 patients

TABLE 5. *Positive findings and false-negative laparoscopies for ovarian cancer by original stage[a]*

Stage	No. cases	Positive	%	No. false negative/ total no.	%
I and II	12	1	8	0/5	
III and IV	9	3	33	3/4	75
Total	21	4	19	3/9	33

[a]Author's data.

had inadequate visualization because of extensive adhesions, and the third patient had only retroperitoneal nodal disease that could not have been identified by laparoscopy. Accordingly, the false-negative rate for laparoscopy for the stage I and stage II patients was 0/5 (0%), the stage III and stage IV patients, 3/4 (75%), and for the entire group, 3/9 (33%).

The remaining 10 ovarian cancer patients in the study underwent laparoscopy: 3 for restaging following recent surgery and 7 for confirmation of clinically suspected recurrence. Disease was identified in 7 of the 10 (70%), and only 1 of the 7 had resectable metastases. This area of restaging and surveillance laparoscopy should prove very rewarding, provided the patients are properly selected with respect to which procedure is performed, laparoscopy or laparotomy.

Reports on the use of laparoscopy as a second-look procedure are appearing more frequently, but the identification of recurrent or residual disease, as in this series, is lower than expected on the basis of information gathered from reports on second-look laparotomy. Of 327 second-look laparoscopies obtained from the literature, only 92 (28%) had positive findings (Table 6). It is not known how many of these 92 patients were resectable, but judging from second-look laparotomy data, the number must be very small. The incidence of false-negative second-look laparos-

TABLE 6. *Positive findings and false-negative second-look laparoscopies, collected series*

Year	Ref.	Patients	Positive	%	No. false negative/ total no.	%
1981	(1)	57	20	35		
1981	(5)	66	24	36	12/22	55
1980	(6)	22	8	36	2/10	20
1980	(7)	62	14	22	3/17	18
1979	(4)	28	3	10	6/18	33
1977	(10)	24	8	33	5/11	45
1976	(11)	47	11	33		
1982	This chapter	21	4	19	3/9	33
	Total	327	92	28	31/87	36

copy in this series is also very high (Table 6). Of 86 patients who underwent a second laparotomy after a negative laparoscopy, 31 (36%) were found to have residual disease missed at laparoscopy. These numbers and the knowledge that recurrence can be identified sometimes only microscopically on random biopsies or in an isolated retroperitoneal node underscore the importance of a formal laparotomy on any patient at high risk for recurrence with a negative second-look laparoscopy. Negative in this context would include cytologic and histologic samples.

Despite the somewhat disappointing results noted above, recent reports by Quinn et al. (7) and Berek et al. (1) indicate that the routine use of cytology at the time of second-look laparoscopy may significantly increase our understanding of the second-look concept. In Quinn's study, there were 48 patients with no gross evidence of tumor at second-look laparoscopy. Cytology was obtained in all patients. Twenty-six of the patients had negative cytology. Of these, 20 (77%) had ceased treatment and were alive and off chemotherapy at least 12 months without evidence of recurrence, 4 (15%) had died of their disease, and 2 (8%) were still being treated. Twenty-two of the 48 patients had positive cytology only, and of these, 12 (55%) were dead and 5 (23%) were still being treated. Only 5 (23%) were alive without evidence of disease and off treatment at least 12 months at the time of this writing. Berek et al. (1) were able to calculate the actuarial survival of 57 ovarian cancer patients who underwent successful laparoscopy 6 months after initiation of adjuvant therapy. The actuarial survival of 37 patients who had negative cytologic and negative gross examination was 80% at 48 months, while there were no survivors at 48 months among 20 patients with positive gross or cytologic findings. Surely these reports should prompt an expanded role for cytology in the laparoscopic surveillance of ovarian cancer patients undergoing adjuvant chemotherapy. It is now an accepted fact that peritoneal cytology should be a routine part of any exploration for gynecologic cancer; this should apply to laparoscopic exploration as well.

CERVICAL CANCER

Although it is known that cervical cancer can produce visceral and peritoneal metastases, this rarely acknowledged pathway of propagation is usually ignored in treatment planning.

We have laparoscopically evaluated 31 patients with squamous-cell carcinoma of the cervix: 22 stage IIb and stage IIIb patients as part of an extended staging work-up during initial pretreatment evaluation and 9 patients for suspected recurrence of cervical cancer at varying intervals of time following treatment. Of the 22 patients laparoscoped for extended staging, 7 (32%) had peritoneal metastases (1 patient with positive cytology only). Of the 15 patients without visceral metastases, 8 underwent an extraperitoneal aortic node dissection and 1 underwent a transperitoneal aortic-node dissection. Four of these patients had positive aortic nodes. The combination of laparoscopy and aortic-node dissection therefore identified 11 of 22 patients (50%) with metastases outside the standard radiation portals (Table 7).

Nine cervical cancer patients underwent laparoscopy for suspected recurrence when other less invasive techniques failed to provide the histologic diagnosis. Three

TABLE 7. *Cervical cancer patients with peritoneal metastases at laparoscopy or positive aortic-node dissection*

	Peritoneal disease			Nodes		Total	
	No.	Positive	%	Positive	%	Positive	%
Staging	22	7	32	4	18	11	50
Surveillance	9	3	33	2	22	5	55
Total	31	10	32	6	19	16	48

of the 9 (33%) had peritoneal disease. Of the 6 patients without peritoneal disease, 1 underwent extraperitoneal aortic-node dissection and 1 had a laparoscopically directed needle biopsy of a large periaortic mass. Both patients had nodal metastases. Therefore, in this small group of patients with suspected recurrent cervical cancer, laparoscopy and aortic-node evaluation identified recurrence in 5 of 9 cases (55%) (Table 7).

The preliminary data indicate that laparoscopy may have some importance as an adjunctive staging procedure for advanced cervical cancer when the usual diagnostic studies, including computerized axial tomography and fine-needle biopsy, do not demonstrate disease outside the standard treatment fields. There have been reports of long-term survivors following aortic radiation therapy for microscopic nodal disease, and therefore it is important to identify and treat such metastases. The same cannot be said for cervical cancer patients with peritoneal implants, since they are all ultimately doomed to fail current treatment methods. For patients with poor prognosis, there is practical merit in considering an accelerated radiation course to control bleeding and pain while conserving valuable time for chemotherapy or other important affairs in anticipation of a downward turn.

OTHER NEOPLASMS

Eleven patients were laparoscoped for other genital or visceral primaries, of which 8 had unresectable intraperitoneal disease and 3 had resectable cancers requiring laparotomy (Table 8). Laparoscopy was clearly beneficial for most of the patients (73%) by obviating the need for laparotomy. Most of the patients were old or medically debilitated, with suspected advanced intraperitoneal disease, and in a sense they were ideal candidates for laparoscopy as a means of providing a histologic diagnosis and assessment of disease volume without the burden of a formal laparotomy.

SUMMARY

When the results of the 92 patients discussed above are measured against the standard of a laparotomy to obtain the same information, 38 of 92 (41%) were spared the risk, expense, and morbidity of the more major procedure (Table 9). In these patients, the laparoscopic findings established an accurate diagnosis and obviated the need for further investigation or surgery. This was especially true for

TABLE 8. *Miscellaneous patients with suspected peritoneal metastases[a]*

Primary cancer	No. cases	Peritoneal disease	%
Endometrial	6	5	83
Vaginal	2	0	
Breast	1	1	
Gastric	1	1	
Mesothelioma	1	1	
Total	11	8	73

[a]Author's data.

the diagnosis of suspected or suspicious pelvic masses and for patients with suspected peritoneal carcinomatosis. The experience reported here with laparoscopy as a second-look procedure for ovarian cancer is similar to that reported by others, and while disappointing from the standpoint of false-negative results, the results will surely improve with better patient selection and the routine use of peritoneal cytology. This limited experience with cervical cancer suggests that laparoscopy may have a role in identifying disease outside the usual treatment portals in patients with advanced disease, especially when combined with routine peritoneal cytology and extraperitoneal aortic-node dissection.

As with any surgical procedure, judgment must be exercized at several levels. Patients should be carefully selected, and the choice between laparotomy and laparoscopy should be made on the basis of the clinical situation, the patient's condition, and the relative merits of each technique and not on the basis of the surgeon's preference for one procedure over another. Technical success or failure in terms of results and complications will depend on surgical experience, skill, and attention to detail. Success in terms of the patient's prognosis will depend on the surgeon's ability to interpret the findings and decide upon a course of action.

It can be said that the medical profession is currently undergoing a technological revolution of unprecedented proportions, which in many respects has produced a

TABLE 9. *Patients spared laparotomy by intercession with laparoscopy*

Primary site	No. cases	Positive	Negative	Patients spared laparotomy	
				No.	%
Cervix	31	8	23	8	26
Ovary	50	22	28	22	44
Other	11	8	3	8	73
Total	92	38	54	38	41

deleterious effect on clinical judgment and physical examination skills, particularly the pelvic examination. It is not at all uncommon to see gynecology patients who have been subjected to many expensive procedures, including pelvic sonography and computerized axial tomography, without the benefit of a prior pelvic examination. Sonographers and tomographers promote their respective instrumentation as the most accurate for diagnosis of pelvic conditions. They offer a percentage likelihood of one diagnosis or another based on films obtained by a technician and interpreted by a physician who in most cases has never examined the patient. Certainly, a pelvic examination is never performed simultaneously to correlate the clinical, sonographic, or radiographic findings. These procedures cannot provide a histologic diagnosis or true assessment of disease volume no matter how experienced the interpreter. Laparoscopy, on the other hand, is safe, simple, fast, and in many cases definitive. Under the direction of an experienced laparoscopist, the procedure becomes almost an extension of the physical examination. While the cost may initially seem high, the information obtained will usually eliminate the need for other expensive nondefinitive procedures and laboratory tests, all of which together far exceed the cost of laparoscopy. For these reasons, I believe laparoscopy should be given due consideration whenever a definitive answer, such as histologic confirmation, is required for treatment planning.

REFERENCES

1. Berek, J. S., Griffiths, C. T., and Leventhal, J. M. (1981): Laparoscopy for second-look evaluation in ovarian cancer. *Obstet. Gynecol.*, 58:192–198.
2. Lacey, C. G. (1976): Laparoscopy. *Obstet. Gynecol.*, 47:625–627.
3. Lacey, C. G., Morrow, C. P., Disaia, P. J., and Lucas, W. E. (1978): Laparoscopy. *Obstet. Gynecol.*, 52:708–712.
4. Mangioni, C., Bolis, G., Molteni, P., and Belloni, C. (1979): Indications, advantages, and limits of laparoscopy in ovarian cancer. *Gynecol. Oncol.*, 7:47–55.
5. Ozols, R. F., Fisher, R. I., Anderson, T., Makuch, R., and Young, R. C. (1981): Peritoneoscopy in the management of ovarian cancer. *Am. J. Obstet. Gynecol.*, 140:611–623.
6. Piver, M. S., Lele, S. B., Barlow, J. J., and Gamarra, M. (1980): Second-look laparoscopy prior to proposed second-look laparotomy. *Obstet. Gynecol.*, 55:571–573.
7. Quinn, M. A., Bishop, G. J., Campbell, J. J., Rodgerson, J., and Pepperell, R. J. (1980): Laparoscopic follow-up of patients with ovarian carcinoma. *Br. J. Obstet. Gynaecol.*, 87:1132–1139.
8. Rosenoff, S. H., Young, R. C., Anderson, T., Bagley, C., Chabner, B., Schein, P. S., Hubbard, S., and DeVita, V. T. (1975): Peritoneoscopy: A valuable staging tool in ovarian carcinoma. *Ann. Intern. Med.*, 83:37–41.
9. Ruddock, J. C. (1937): Peritoneoscopy. *Surg. Gynecol. Obstet.*, 65:623–639.
10. Smith, G. W., Day, T. G., Jr., and Smith, J. P. (1977): The use of laparoscopy to determine the results of chemotherapy for ovarian cancer. *J. Reprod. Med.*, 18:257–260.
11. Spinelli, R., Luini, A., Pizzetti, P., and De Palo, G. M. (1976): Laparoscopy in staging and restaging of 95 patients with ovarian carcinoma. *Tumori*, 62:493–502.

Recent Clinical Developments in Gynecologic Oncology, edited by C. Paul Morrow, et al. Raven Press, New York © 1983.

Management of Pain in Gynaecological Cancer Patients

Hugh Raftery

St. Laurence's Hospital, Terenure, Dublin 6, Ireland

Peripheral-nerve pain, however, is commonly seen. It usually is caused by the compression of lumbar or sacral nerve trunks by a tumour, either at the pelvic brim or in the substance of the psoas muscle. It is common with stage 4 cancer of the cervix but can also occur with tumours of the corpus uteri, ovaries, or vulva with advanced glandular spread. Peripheral-nerve compression pain is characterised by its referral to the peripheral distribution of the nerve, lack of tenderness in the painful area, and very effective relief by opiates. Such pain also may be caused by direct invasion of nerve trunks by tumours, which may be suspected by the greater intensity of the pain, by the potentiation of pain by movement, and by the greater doses of opiates required to achieve less relief.

In this chapter, I will discuss the principles of pain assessment and describe the main management techniques.

PATIENT ASSESSMENT

In assessing the patient's pain, it is useful to remember that there are three main ways that pain may be generated, giving rise to three types of pain: central pain, peripheral-nerve compression pain, and pain as a result of damage to peripheral tissues.

Central pain rarely arises in gynaecological tumours, and if it does it indicates that the tumour has spread to the central nervous system. Central pain is recognized by its deep boring nature, and in gynaecological practice it would indicate cerebral or spinal-cord secondary tumours.

Peripheral-nerve pain, however, is commonly seen. It usually is caused by the compression of lumbar or sacral nerve trunks by a tumour, either at the pelvic brim or in the substance of the psoas muscle. It is common with stage 4 cancer of the cervix but can also occur with tumours of the corpus uteri, ovaries, or vulva with advanced glandular spread. Peripheral-nerve compression pain is characterised by its referral to the peripheral distribution of the nerve, lack of tenderness in the painful area, and very effective relief by opiates. Such pain also may be caused by direct invasion of nerve trunks by tumours, which may be suspected by the greater intensity of the pain, by the potentiation of pain by movement, and by the greater doses of opiates required to achieve less relief.

The third mechanism of pain generation is engendered by damage to peripheral tissues with the consequent release of bradykinin, serotonin, and the like, the further secretion of prostaglandins, and the recognition of a tender painful area. Intense pain and tenderness at the site of the tumour are characteristic. The nerve supply of such tender masses may not be very clear and may well be mixed somatic and autonomic.

Assessment of the pain on the basis of these three mechanisms is the first step toward selecting the best approach to management.

In the management of any symptom, it is important that the physician be certain that the identified disease is indeed the cause of the symptom. It is also necessary that he know if some other pathology is present and if the patient is undergoing any other treatment, particularly the drugs involved.

Having established the patient's background and having conducted a physical examination, the physician is now ready for the next important assessment, namely, the patient's reaction to the existing condition. It is very difficult to treat a patient for pain if it is not possible to talk about the cause of the pain, what can and cannot be done, what unwanted outcomes may follow treatment, and why these may be more acceptable than the natural progression of the disease. The patient's understanding of and insight into the nature of the disease are important factors in her acceptance of pain relief rather than cure. A state of trust should exist between the physician and patient, and this should not be destroyed by the establishment of unrealistic treatment goals.

In making a psychological assessment of the patient, it is rarely necessary to engage in elaborate psychological scoring systems. It has been shown that in most patients suffering from chronic pain, anxiety and neurotic behaviour will revert to normal upon the establishment of an adequate pain-relief programme (1–5). In the few patients requiring treatment for anxiety and depression, time should be set aside for more detailed analysis, counselling, and treatment.

If treatment goals are realistic and the limitations on life-style are accepted, then the prospects of relative comfort until death are good.

PAIN MANAGEMENT

Four factors play a role in pain management, and the relative importance of each factor will have been indicated by the preliminary assessment. The four factors are:

1. pain signal interruption,
2. pain suppression by various drug combinations,
3. attention to coincidental symptoms, such as constipation, urinary or chest infections, dehydration, or starvation,
4. psychological support.

Signal Interruption

If a clear-cut peripheral-nerve referred pain is the principal complaint, perhaps owing to nerve trunk compression by stage 4 cancer of the cervix at the pelvic side wall, then a simple subarachnoid alcohol nerve-root block will provide considerable relief. Subarachnoid alcohol or phenol nerve-block injections are useful; they are simple procedures that can produce substantial pain relief for periods of 1 to 2 months in suitable patients. Favourable indications for the use of such a procedure are that the tumour compress rather than invade the nerve trunks, that the pain history be short, and that there be no opiate addiction. Contraindications are that the tumour is invasive or that bone involvement has occurred.

The technique of alcohol subarachnoid block is very simple. The patient is positioned on the pain-free side, with the segment to be blocked highest. A fine lumbar puncture needle is introduced into the subarachnoid space, preferably off centre to the painful side. The patient is tilted forward and 0.1 ml alcohol is introduced, which should produce paraesthesias in the target area. Having confirmed correct placement, additional 0.2 ml alcohol is introduced and after 3 min another 0.2 ml. If more than two roots require neurolysis, it is better to carry out separate needle punctures at two spaced intervals rather than to attempt to float the alcohol. It is also necessary that an adequate dose of alcohol be used, since the incidence of incomplete block and the early recurrence of pain are greater with lower doses. However, larger doses should not be used, since this could lead to excessive motor loss.

The technique for phenol neurolysis is similar, except that since the solution is hyperbaric, that is, it tends to sink, the patient is placed on the painful side and the 6% phenol in glycerine is layered from above. I have found that alcohol provides more effective pain relief in a higher proportion of patients and that the incidence of neuritis and dysaesthesia is similar.

If the pain is more generalised, as with generalised peritoneal spread of ovarian cancer, the splanchnic nervous relay system is involved. This too can be dulled by a relatively simple injection technique at the level of the coeliac plexus. This is done by a posterior paravertebral approach to the anterior surface of the first lumbar vertebra preferably with the assistance of X-ray images; 4 ml alcohol injected into each side is a highly effective anaesthetic for the peritoneal cavity.

Other methods of signal interruption include radio-frequency heat lesioning either of nerve trunks at the intervertebral foramen or of the anterolateral tracts by per-cutaneous cervical cordotomy.

In theory, interruption of nerve pathways between the diseased area and the central nervous system should result in complete loss of pain. However, this rarely is the case in practice. The reasons for this are not always apparent, but they must include the basic inefficiency of neurolytic injections, the progressive nature of the disease process, and possibly the rerouting of the pain signal around the blocked nerve. This is not necessarily bad. The basic inefficiency of the procedure means that the motor and sensory losses are also incomplete, so the disability following the first nerve block is not great. What I seek to achieve from a nerve block is to simplify and render more effective the drug management of pain.

Use of Drugs

The management of pain in cancer patients essentially involves the correct use of drugs in the vast majority of cases, and all other procedures are directed at facilitating this.

A number of guidelines are useful in the administration of pain-killing drugs:

1. Since the problem is continuous, the medication must be continuous, that is, the next dose of analgesic must be given before the pain returns.

2. The medication should correlate with the pain mechanism. This means that anti-inflammatory drugs should be used for peripheral-injury pain, opiates for nerve-damage pain, and anticonvulsants for central pain. In practice, the problem is rarely simple, and drug combinations are often required.

3. Mood-enhancing drugs, such as tricyclic antidepressants or benzodiazepines, may be required and indeed may reduce the effective dosage of analgesics.

4. Common side effects, such as constipation, nausea, and anorexia, should be recognised and steps taken to alleviate them.

It may be pertinent to briefly discuss the use of opiates and anti-inflammatory analgesics. It is characteristic of cancer pain that it is continuous and unrelenting and not relieved by such factors as change in posture, the time of day, or food. In fact, it is only relieved by analgesics, frequently very effectively. Since the pain is continuous, the medication must also be continuous and preferably administered by mouth. Absorption can take up to 1 hr, and consequently the dosage must be titrated against the patient's requirements and administered on a time scale determined by the length of action of the drugs in a particular patient. A 2-hr drug is given every 2 hr, a 4-hr drug, every 4 hr, and so on. While the correct oral dose is being determined, it is usually necessary to supplement it with intramuscular injections, preferably of the same drugs. I favour the use of morphine. It is readily available, inexpensive, effective by mouth, sufficiently long acting, and effectively controls pain. The disadvantages of nausea, constipation, and tolerance can be managed, particularly when they are anticipated. Tolerance usually builds up during the first 2 weeks of use, whereupon dose levels should be stabilised, usually at twice the amount of the starting dose but sometimes more. Thus morphine should be given orally every 4, 5, or 6 hr, depending on the patient, in a dose sufficient to ease the pain. When necessary, this dose should be increased until a steady state is reached. If antinauseants are required to suppress vomiting, they can usually be withdrawn after 1 week, when steady blood levels are achieved. Oral morphine is best administered in solution, since this ensures absorption. Tablets are also available, including a recently marketed slow-release tablet. In my experience, slow-release tablets are not always absorbed satisfactorily, but when they are, the twice a day administration is very convenient.

When the pain is caused by both peripheral damage and nerve compression, which is quite common, mixed analgesic management is necessary, consisting of antiinflammatory medication and opiates. Here again, it is desirable to achieve twice a day dosage, and there are some antiinflammatory drugs available now that are potent prostaglandin inhibitors with 12-hr sustained action. Such drugs as Difusinal, Peroxicam, or Finclofenac can enhance the effect of the morphine by relieving the inflammatory aspects of the pain.

Other drugs may be required but should not be added on a routine basis. It is not at all surprising that because of the persistence of chronic pain and the terminal nature of the illness patients often become neurotic and depressed. Control of the pain and a firm commitment to maintain the control will go a long way toward relieving the depression and may be all the medication that is required. However, tricyclic antidepressant drugs can help and work well in combination with morphine; 50 mg amitriptyline nightly is usually sufficient.

Other Aspects of Pain Management

Another aspect of drug management necessitates a look at the whole patient. Other causes of pain and discomfort should be treated or alleviated, e.g., superficial infections, dehydration, constipation, urinary retention, and even starvation. These problems usually do not arise in hospitals but may in domiciliary practice.

It is important that the patient make her peace with God, family, and friends and, in turn, receive support from her church, family, and physicians.

Only a small number of patients who die of cancer do so in severe pain. When advancing cancer does cause pain, it usually indicates peripheral-nerve involvement. Such pain can be a severe test of therapy and demands the full attention of the attending physician. The various psychotherapy techniques used in chronic pain management have little place in this field. What patients need is practical pain relief, which can be achieved by a combination of neurolytic procedures and the careful use of analgesics in doses suitable to the clinical need and their therapeutic capabilities.

Life expectancy is short, usually a matter of months. Insight into the condition varies from patient to patient. Emotional support for patient and family is necessary, and a most important part of this support is the assurance that pain relief will always be available. The fear is not of death but of death alone and in pain. This need not and should not happen.

REFERENCES

1. Bond, M. R. (1976): Pain and personality in cancer patients. In: *Advances in Pain Research and Therapy, Vol. 1*, edited by J. J. Bonica and D. Albe Fessard, pp. 311–316. Raven Press, New York.
2. Evans, R. J., and Mackay, I. M. (1972): Subarachnoid phenol nerve blocks for relief of pain in advanced malignancy. *Can. J. Surg.*, 15(1):50–53.
3. Lifshitz, S., Debacker, L. J., and Buchsbaum, H. J. (1976): Subarachnoid phenol block for pain relief in gynecological malignancy. *Obstet. Gynecol.*, 48(3):316–320.
4. Renaer, M., and Guzinski, G. M. (1978): Pain in gynaecological practice. *Pain*, 5(4):305–331.
5. Sternbach, R. A., and Timmermans, G. (1975): Personality changes associated with reduction in pain. *Pain*, 1:177–181.

Recent Clinical Developments in Gynecologic Oncology, edited by C. Paul Morrow, et al. Raven Press, New York © 1983.

Terminal Care of the Gynaecological Cancer Patient

Michael J. O'Halloran

Saint Luke's Hospital, Rathgar, Dublin 6, Ireland

Most of the efforts today in the field of oncology are directed at prevention, early diagnosis, and improved survival. In the field of gynaecological cancer, while these three aspects are clearly identified and a reduction in the death rate from uterine cancer has been achieved, there still remain patients requiring terminal care. There are two types of cancer patients requiring such care: the patient who develops recurrent malignant disease that is incurable and the patient who has incurable disease at first presentation.

Physicians feel it is their responsibility to restore patients to health when they succumb to illness. When a patient develops recurrent malignant disease that is incurable, physicians find it difficult to accept that they have failed. However, it is important to understand that a genuine effort was made to cure the patient from the outset, and consequently the failure to do so should be acceptable to the physician because the attempt itself brings a certain kind of fulfillment.

The patient who presents with incurable disease at first attendance is unlikely to experience a reasonable interval of freedom from symptoms, and so the mental attitude of such a patient is likely to be focused on death as the eventual outcome.

In the course of treating the patient with incurable disease, physicians have the opportunity to learn and study the patient's personality and family, and when the terminal stage is approached, the management will have acquired many useful strategies, which can be incorporated in the treatment. In caring for terminal patients, the art of medicine must take over when the science of medicine has failed.

Many terminally ill patients develop infection, while some develop sepsis. A lowered immunocompetence interferes with the host's ability to respond normally to infection. However, specimens of sputum, blood, and urine and swabs from discharging sinuses and ulcers taken for culturing and to determine sensitivity can contribute to the determination of which antibiotic therapy is appropriate and which medications are unsuitable.

If blood transfusions are required, there may be some difficulty in crossmatching such patients because of the presence of an antibody that complicates the crossmatch. The administration of cortisone can often temporarily suppress the antibody.

The symptoms that terminally ill gynaecological patients complain of vary, depending on the original primary site of the tumour.

MAJOR SYMPTOMS OF TERMINAL PATIENTS

Pain. Pain can be controlled with adequate analgesics, with or without sedatives, and it is important to continually change the preparations until a suitable regime has been achieved. The principal goal of the physician is to achieve 24-hr freedom from pain and a state where the patient remains comfortable during the day and sleeps undisturbed through the night. An oral drug regime is desirable, so that injections are reduced to a minimum. Adequate drug dosage is essential at this stage. Morhpine sulphate combined with dextroamphetamine in an oral liquid preparation can provide adequate pain relief and at the same time reduce drowsiness. Occasionally, as with carcinoma of the cervix, pelvic and lower limb pain may be due to involvement of the nerve sheath by neoplastic growth, and a nerve block may be more beneficial for some patients, especially when combined with other drug therapy. Bone metastases are uncommon, but not unknown, with gynaecological cancer and, if present, are treated by radiotherapy and drug medication.

Bladder. Incontinence or retention of urine is generally adequately cared for by an in-dwelling catheter. However, if catheterisation is not practical, the patient's general condition is reasonably good, and the life expectancy is a few months, then ureterostomy should be considered.

Bowel. Intestinal obstruction is best treated by conservative measures, such as intravenous fluids and suction, since attempts at colostomy may lead to further complications.

Ascites. Ascites and pleural effusions are more frequently associated with ovarian tumours, and adequate drainage and instillation of tetracycline or cytotoxic drugs into the cavities may provide reasonable relief and control.

Oedema. Oedema of the lower limbs may be the result of tumour masses in the pelvis or recurrence of growth in the groin following previous block dissection. Rest and elevation of the lower limbs is the only worthwhile procedure that temporarily reduces oedema. Drugs have proved to be disappointing.

Fistula. Vaginal fistula formation between the bladder or rectum as a result of direct growth or a treatment complication may require ureterostomy or colostomy.

Cachexia. Cachexia in the cancer patient is a complex metabolic problem involving all systems to one degree or another. All the abnormalities need appropriate medications, and at times a central venous line allows for easier correction and nursing while least disturbing the patient. If progressive emaciation becomes apparent, it can be a disturbing sign to the patient and relatives.

OTHER ASPECTS

Other important aspects that play a role in terminal-care management include the personality of the patient and relatives and the relationship between the patient and physician and members of the supporting medical and paramedical team. It is important that the patient's care and interests are given priority at all times. It is essential that a member of the caring team is always available for discussions with the patient and the next of kin. Unfortunately, some physicians are unable to handle their patients' emotional problems and transfer this responsibility to junior members of the staff. When the patient must attend a cancer hospital especially dealing with recurrent or incurable cancer, this may often be the first indication to the patient that she has cancer, and at this initial counselling it is necessary to express genuine interest in the patient's symptoms and reassure her of relieving them. It is essential that discussions with the patient are never hurried and show that the physician is interested in what the patient has to say. Once a good line of communication has been established, the physician should strive to divert the patient from thoughts of cancer. As time elapses, most patients recognise the seriousness of their condition, and if trust has been developed between physician and patient, she will accept the varying symptoms as long as she is convinced of the physician's readiness to help.

WHAT TO TELL THE PATIENT

There is no question that the patient is entitled to be told the truth, and most works written on the subject concur in this. However, there are some physicians who in dealing with the terminal-cancer patient have regretted telling some patients of their impending death. It is my practice to study the patient and her relatives over a period of time, and having assessed their commitment and responsibility and their real desire to know the facts, I first tell the relatives and then, with their consent or request, the patient, if in my opinion the patient is desirous of a truthful answer.

A matter that is seldom discussed is the personality of the attending physician. Unfortunately, some members of the medical profession are unsuited to deal with what can be more of an emotional problem than a medical symptom.

In conclusion, anxiety, grief, depression, anger, and denial are the most normal emotional reactions in the terminal-cancer patient. All of these can be resolved to some extent by the trust and confidence the patient has in those who care for her.

Subject Index

Subject Index